Ethical Dilemmas

in Reproduction

Ethical Dilemmas

in Reproduction

Edited by

F. Shenfield

University College London
London, UK

and

C. Sureau

Institut Theramex
Paris, France

The Parthenon Publishing Group

International Publishers in Medicine, Science & Technology

A CRC PRESS COMPANY
BOCA RATON   LONDON   NEW YORK   WASHINGTON, D.C.

Published in the USA by
The Parthenon Publishing Group
345 Park Avenue South, 10th Floor
New York, NY 10010, USA

Published in the UK and Europe by
The Parthenon Publishing Group
23–25 Blades Court, Deodar Road
London, SW15 2NU, UK

Library of Congress Cataloging-in-Publication Data
Ethical dilemmas in reproduction / [edited by] F. Shenfield, C. Sureau
          p. ; cm.
    Rev. ed. of : Ethical dilemmas in assisted reproduction.
    Includes bibliographical references and index.
    ISBN 1-84214-093-0 (alk. paper)
        1. Human reproduction—Moral and ethical aspects. 2. Human
reproductive technology—Moral and ethical aspects. I. Shenfield,
Françoise. II. Sureau, Claude. III. Ethical dilemmas in assisted
reproduction.
        [DNLM: 1. Reproductive Techniques. 2. Ethics, Clinical.
3. Reproduction. WQ208E844 2002]
    RG133.5+   2002018349

British Library Cataloguing in Publication Data
Shenfield, Francoise
    Ethical dilemmas in reproduction
    1. Human reproductive technology – Moral and ethical aspects
    I. Title II. Sureau, Claude
    176
    ISBN 1-84214-093-0

Typeset by Martin Lister Publishing Services, Carnforth, UK

Printed and bound by Bookcraft (Bath) Ltd., Midsomer Norton, UK

Contents

Foreword

This second book on ethical issues in reproduction, edited by Françoise Shenfield and Claude Sureau, will be welcomed by all physicians, scientists, infertile couples, ethicists and thinking members of society in general who are challenged by so many of the contentious issues arising out of the practice of assisted reproductive techniques today.

This volume deals in a very lucid way with many of the fundamental issues that we, as providers of treatment, face in caring for our infertile patients. As clinicians and scientists, we are always being asked to advise couples on their fertility treatment options: for example, when one or other partner is about to start cancer therapy; when one or other partner is HIV positive or if a couple are concerned about the chances of high-order multiple pregnancy. It is impossible for us as caring individuals not to be strongly influenced by a couple's particular needs, and yet there may be a conflict between what we believe may be the best option for them and what is 'right' or 'ethical' to society. Most important is the consideration of the welfare of any child. It is possible for us, clinicians in particular, to become so 'wrapped up' in what we perceive to be best for the couple, that we do not see the 'wider picture'. A good example is in agreeing to transfer multiple embryos to a woman in the hope that the chance of achieving a single healthy baby might be improved. If, however, triplets are born, of whom one or more may be handicapped, the mother may become profoundly depressed and the husband may walk out on the marriage. This would not be an outcome that the well-intentioned clinician would have wished for his patients, their children or society in general.

We must also ask ourselves if it is right to offer a young woman about to start anticancer therapy the option to freeze some of her oocytes or ovarian tissue in the hope that in the future we may be able to use them to help her to have a child. The technology does not yet allow use of ovarian tissue; however, if we do not counsel couples and explain their options, without trying to raise their hopes unreasonably, we have failed them at their time of greatest need. Moreover, we will also have failed them if the technology does then become available in the future.

The ethical issues covered in this volume are reviewed at a most appropriate time. All of the subjects covered in the nine chapters address ethical issues that have featured extensively in the medical, scientific and lay literature in these first 2 years of the 21st century. I am sure that this excellent book, written by authors celebrated in their fields and edited by two of the best known figures in this particular area of ethics, will be avidly read by many clinicians and scientists, as well as patients. I also strongly believe that it should be read by the 'average man in the street', who represents society at large, and who really should be interested in these fascinating issues that challenge us today.

Peter R. Brinsden, MB, FRCOG
Bourn Hall Clinic
Bourn, Cambridge, UK

Preface

This book is in the spirit and follows the previous joint effort of the editors when essential subjects like the ethics of embryo research or of sex selection were discussed. Since then, scientific facts and social attitudes have changed and progressed. Nothing is static, even in France where both the Conseil d'État and different government members have publicly stated that it is time to go on with embryo research, especially considering the exciting promises of the therapeutic techniques from stem cells, including embryo stem cells (SC).

Some new techniques are too experimental to discuss in this book, as for instance the removal of fragments from embryos, the artificial induction of meiosis, or the reproductive problems of homosexuals or transsexuals. But there was a need for another book, with a very similar title to that edited in 1997. The principles of analysis are the same, an intellectual logical appraisal of why one feels that some of the techniques stemming from assisted reproductive technology (ART) may be right or wrong, at the personal as well as the social level. This is where ethics and legal analysis are both important, as they reflect the eternal dialectics between democratic societies and their citizens. Thus an analysis of recent cases in negligence after fetal damage helps to revisit the status of the fetus in relation to the child to be. In a similar fashion, the stem cell debate serves to revisit the question of the status of the embryo, and the way to treat it with the respect due to its human quality. But the fact that most embryos are created in ART in order that they become a fetus and then hopefully a child is the important feature of the chapter concerning the ills of multiple pregnancy.

The new possibility of oocyte and ovarian tissue cryopreservation raises the issue of insurance-taking by modern women to preserve their fertility: Wybo Dondorp addresses this in 'Freezing the hands of time: fertility insurance for healthy women'. It may be argued that here we leave therapeutic necessity for another realm, that of social contingency. However, the techniques may be new, but the questions are not. They revolve around sex equality (as men have for long been able to preserve their sperm for future reproduction), the impact of new technologies, and the welfare of the child thus conceived. The same technology may also be used for the preservation of the fertility of cancer sufferers. Always a poignant dilemma, it is perhaps even more so in the case of young patients, children and adolescents, raising acute legal questions of consent as well as ethical dilemmas intrinsic to youth and the responsibility we have towards them singly and collectively.

As for Guido Pennings, he addresses 'the moral responsibility of the physician for providing infertility treatment to HIV positive people', raising the issues of discrimination and selection of patients. Again, not a new question in our field, but one completely modified by the worst new disease to have erupted in the last century, still taking a huge toll internationally in the new millennium. With Inge Liebaers, he tackles another new dilemma, raised by preimplantation genetic diagnosis (PGD) with a difference, that of 'Creating a child to save another: HLA matching of siblings through preimplantation genetic diagnosis'. Since this event, described a year ago, more events of the same nature have been published, generally called preimplantation genetic selection (or screening; PGS), a matter discussed in our previous book. Selection is a historically charged word, and it may be asked whether it can also be used in a positive, life enhancing fashion and be given a new respectability. The other problem raised is whether such creation of a child for a benefit to another is compatible with the Kantian categorical imperative or not using a person merely as means to another. Finally it rekindles the perennial question of the intrinsic value of life, as alluded to in the chapter concerning wrongful life and death.

This book is a practical offering to our fellow practitioners to help articulate and solve some of those questions asked in many, if not all, fields of medicine: life and quality of life, in this specialty where we have the privilege to help create a new life.

And when we help create it with the best intentions, the results may be unexpected, as the anguish shown by some of the children of gametes donation who claim that secrets and anonymity have deprived them of a part of their identity (Juliet Tizzard). This is another question revolving around essence (oneself, one's identity) rather than just existence, and quality of life.

Finally, there are wonderful hopes from techniques linked to reproduction, and in particular those linked to cloning. In the chapter 'Cloning: reproductive, therapeutic or not at all?' Françoise Shenfield discusses more issues which take us back to the ontological status of the embryo, and the subject of egg donation. We face again the dilemma of balancing the benefit we may gather from any new technique, a utilitarian approach, with the principle of taking essential questions like the respect of the embryo as a human entity into account. These are exciting questions, everyday questions not only for practitioners and their patients, but also for society at large as witnessed by the daily media interest. We hope that readers will find them as interesting as the editors and authors do, and that this book will offer a few tools for anyone interested in challenging their own moral reasoning, as we were.

F. Shenfield
C. Sureau
February 2002

Bibliography

Shenfield F, Sureau C, eds. *Ethical Dilemmas in Assisted Reproduction*. London: Parthenon Publishing, 1997

List of Principal Contributors

Dr Jean Cohen
Director, Centre de Stérilité à l'Hôpital de Sèvres
Paris, France

Dr Wybo J Dondorp
Gezondheidsraad (Health Council of the Netherlands)
The Hague, The Netherlands

Prof Dr Inge Liebaers
Free University Brussels
Brussels, Belgium

Dr Guido Pennings
Free University Brussels
Brussels, Belgium

Dr Françoise Shenfield
University College London
London, UK

Prof Claude Sureau
Institut Theramex
Paris, France

Juliet Tizzard
Director, Progress Educational Trust
London, UK

1

Freezing the hands of time: fertility insurance for healthy women?

W.J. Dondorp

INTRODUCTION

In a popular book on modern reproductive technologies (*How to get Pregnant with the New Technology*), the American gynecologist S. J. Silber speaks of cryopreservation of ovarian tissue as a new solution for women who at 35 have no permanent partner but still want children: 'you can save your eggs for later'[1]. The Internet site of the Genetics & IVF Institute in Fairfax, VA (USA) already offers this intervention to 'normal reproductive age women anticipating delayed childbearing' as part of an approved experimental program[2]. The solution proposed to these women is a spin-off of technology developed in a medical context: cryopreservation of ovarian tissue as 'fertility insurance' for (young) women who, as a result of medical intervention or disease, are at risk of losing their fertility. Whether it will really be possible for them to secure their reproductive potential in this way is not yet clear. Freezing the tissue is one thing, using it for reproduction after thawing is something quite different. Although the first human auto-transplants have been reported, there has not yet been a pregnancy that used oocytes from cryopreserved ovarian tissue. Animal studies, however, suggest that this method of fertility insurance will be technically possible. Once this has been shown to be a reliable, safe technology, it is not inconceivable that women may indeed request its application to protect their reproductive options from the natural loss of fertility from aging ovaries.

In a recent advisory report on future developments in assisted reproductive technology (ART), the Health Council of the Netherlands draws attention to this possibility as 'fertility insurance for non-medical reasons'. The council observes that 'it is questionable whether this is a desirable development'[3]. Others have taken a similar position, using such phrases as 'moral dilemma'[4]. Exactly what makes this a dilemma is unclear. In this essay I will summarize the state of biomedical science in this area and examine the relevant arguments for evaluating the dilemma.

CRYOPRESERVATION OF OOCYTES AND OVARIAN TISSUE AS FERTILITY INSURANCE

Cryopreservation of sperm from men in danger of losing their fertility from needed medical procedures (chemotherapy, radiation) is an established practice. In recent years the availability of intracytoplasmic sperm injection (ICSI) has considerably improved the chances for successful future use of cryopreserved sperm, as sperm quality and quantity are no longer limiting factors[5]. For women, there is no real equivalent to this, because IVF using frozen-thawed oocytes is not yet a realistic option[6]. Sometimes embryos are created and then cryopreserved as fertility insurance for couples when the woman requires medical treatment that poses a threat to her fertility[7,8], but this is a questionable alternative for various reasons (practical, emotional, medical and moral).

Cryopreservation of oocytes

Because mature oocytes are in a vulnerable developmental phase, freezing and thawing can easily disturb the oocyte's internal organization and cause chromosomal damage[9]. Although the first clinical experiments were reported in the late eighties, very few children have been born from cryopreserved oocytes. Some researchers believe that more favorable results can be expected from newly developed freeze and thaw protocols and from the use of ICSI for fertilization[10]. Furthermore, cryopreservation of mature oocytes is a far from ideal method of fertility insurance. To obtain a sufficient quantity of oocytes for freezing requires the use of a burdensome, time-consuming and (for cancer patients) sometimes contraindicated hormone treatment. Moreover, girls who have not yet reached puberty could not be helped with this technology. A better option is cryopreservation of immature (but full grown and 'meiotically competent') oocytes that can be recovered through transvaginal puncture. It is biologically plausible that oocytes at this stage of their development (prophase I) are far less sensitive to damage from freezing and thawing than are fully mature oocytes[5]. Freezing of immature oocytes, however, would not be worthwhile if they cannot be brought to maturity *in vitro*. Research on the optimal conditions for *in vitro* maturation of human oocytes (IVM) is promising because of the great potential benefit it could bring to IVF treatment. Although clinical experiments have resulted in pregnancies and births, the developmental viability of embryos created from IVM remains disappointing[11]. The results of animal studies also raise concerns about the safety of clinical applications[3]. Whether the combination of cryopreservation and IVM would constitute an effective, safe method for ensuring fertility is still very unclear. It is obvious, moreover, that the quantity of oocytes that can be harvested per cycle would be a limiting factor. If time allows for no more than one puncture, as may be the case in the context of cancer treatment, the 'insurance' obtained from cryopreserving those oocytes would be limited to just a few IVF or ICSI cycles. In view of the still meager chances of success per cycle, using these techniques to ensure future child-bearing is very uncertain.

Cryopreservation of ovarian tissue

An approach to address this limitation was proposed in the early nineties by the group of the British researcher R. G. Gosden (Leeds). They suggested that cryopreservation of ovarian tissue obtained through biopsy or oophorectomy could preserve hundreds or even thousands of oocytes for future use – and this would be performed during a phase of their development (primordial follicles) in which they are relatively well able to resist the damage of freezing and thawing[12]. After autotransplantation a woman would be able to re-use these follicles for reproductive purposes, possibly without any need to undergo IVF treatment[13,14]. As has been shown in several animal studies, follicles surviving cryopreservation and transplantation retain their developmental potential. In immunodeficient mice, long-term oocyte growth has been demonstrated in human ovarian tissue xenotransplants[15]. Moreover, in studies using rodents and sheep (where the ovaries are physiologically closer to those of humans) long-term fertility was re-established after autotransplantation of previously frozen tissue, leading to normal pregnancies and healthy offspring[16–19].

Autotransplantation of ovarian tissue is possible both where the tissue had previously been removed (orthotopic) and elsewhere in the body (heterotopic). As yet, there is no firm consensus about which site would be preferable. Although orthotopic transplantation, in principle, would allow for subsequent natural conception, for technical and practical reasons (better chances of successful transplantation, better accessibility) heterotopic transplantation may be chosen[14,20]. If this option is invoked, restoration of ovarian function no longer includes natural conception, but it may entail the prospect of (supported) oocyte maturation in the transplant. Thus, for a few years, this would allow the possibility of IVF treatment using an individual's own oocytes. The duration of the recovery would depend on the size of the functional stock of oocytes in the transplant. The likelihood for sustained recovery of ovarian function is greatest in young women and girls[21]. An upper age limit of 35–38 has been proposed for successful experimental cryopreservation of ovarian tissue, as the intervention would be probably useless in women who are older[22,23]. Only a few cases of human ovarian autotransplantation have been reported up to now, and these include both orthotopic and heterotopic grafting. As yet, there have been no reports of pregnancy or long-term restoration of fertility[24,25]. Worldwide, ovarian tissue has been frozen from an unknown number of women for possible future reproductive use.

Autografting, xenografting, in vitro *culture*

As a method for ensuring fertility, the sequence of cryopreservation and autotransplantation of ovarian tissue may seem to have important advantages. Even apart from its greater yield, this method addresses two of the persistent problems of the current alternatives – the sensitivity of mature oocytes to damage from freezing and thawing, and, if immature oocytes are frozen, the need to bring them to full maturation *in vitro*. A further advantage of cryopreservation and autotransplantation is that re-establishment of ovarian function would not only re-establish fertility, but would restore hormonal balance as well. In the cases reported so far, menopausal complaints were the primary reason for transplantation. When applied in cancer patients, the main disadvantage of this technology is the risk that any malignant cells in the transplant might lead to a recurrence of the cancer[26,27]. This risk depends on the type of cancer, its stage and degree of activity[28,29]. If such risk contraindicates autotransplantation, xenotransplantation that uses an animal to incubate the transplanted oocytes could be considered[9,20,30]. It is, however, not yet clear whether this would be a realistic option. The possible success of this technique will depend on the outcome of further evaluation of the risk of cross-species transmission of pathogens attendant on xenotransplantation[31]. A second alternative that has been suggested is isolation of the primordial follicles from the tissue after thawing to grow and mature the oocytes *in vitro*[5,30,32]. If it were possible to do this, from the perspective of making most efficient use of the limited supply of oocytes, this would be the best option by far. Until now, complete *in vitro* growth from the primordial stage has only been achieved in mice, leaving the application to humans far in the future[33]. Judging from the time needed *in vivo*, this technique would require a culture period of 6–7 months, with the optimal conditions not yet known. Nevertheless, some researchers are optimistic[9,20].

Potential applications

The literature mentions three potential applications, each as a response to a different threat to female fertility: medical intervention (iatrogenic), disease (pathologic), and aging (natural loss of fertility)[23].

Iatrogenic loss of fertility

This category includes patients (women and girls) who need to undergo chemotherapy or radiation for cancer. The amount of damage depends on the dose and nature of the treatment and on the age of the woman. Recovery of cyclicity is more often found in younger women, but even they are still at a higher risk of premature menopause[34]. Radiation damage may be limited through shielding or transposition of the ovaries[35]. The benefit of ovarian suppression as a protective measure against damage from chemotherapy is still under discussion[36]. Ensuring fertility through cryo-preservation of ovarian tissue could be an additional protective measure. Furthermore, this category also includes women requiring long-term chemotherapy for treatment of diseases other than cancer (for instance autoimmune diseases) or who stand to lose one or both of their ovaries through surgical intervention. Iatrogenic loss of fertility from gender transformation surgery should also be included here[37]. Cryopreservation of ovarian tissue would offer trans-sexual men (female-to-male) the prospect of being able to have children that are genetically their own. This situation, however, poses further limitations to the possibility of using the frozen reserve for future reproduction. Not only will it be necessary to grow and mature the follicles completely *in vitro* or in a host animal (because autotransplantation after gender assignment is not an option), but transformation surgery also means that another person (female partner or surrogate mother) will have to bear the pregnancy.

Pathologic loss of fertility

Premature ovarian failure (POF) is the loss of ovarian function before or at the age of 40, despite normal puberty and development up to then. The loss of function is related to the premature depletion of the woman's follicular reserve, and its occurrence is generally acute. After that, reproductive options are limited to IVF using donor oocytes. In most cases the cause of premature failure is unknown (idiopathic POF); where there is a known cause, it comes about either through medical intervention (iatrogenic, as discussed above) or is associated with infectious disease, protein shortage, cytogenetic anomaly, genetic mutation, or auto-immune disease[38,39]. Women known to be at greater risk for POF from disease or an associated condition, or because they are from a family with a higher incidence of this would (theoretically) be able to protect themselves against loss of fertility through timely ovarian tissue freezing[23,40]. The difficulty is that there are no precise indicators for POF nor the time frame when it might take place.

Natural loss of fertility

Besides iatrogenic and pathologic loss of fertility, the third threat to which cryopreservation of ovarian tissue may be an answer, is that of time: the process of follicular depletion which renders women infertile in their early forties and ten years later causes menopause. The greater life expectancy of modern women has not resulted in an extension of their reproductive lifespan – it has even made it comparatively shorter[41]. This effect becomes more pressing when it is linked to a later average maternity age. In the

5

Netherlands the average age at which women have their first child increased from 27.6 in 1990 to 29.1 in 1999[42]. A similar tendency is apparent in many other countries, including the UK. One important element governing this is the degree to which women are able to combine their desire to have children with their other aspirations for education, career, and (partner) relationships[43]. As a result, a growing group of women require medical assistance for reproduction, often resulting in an unfulfilled desire to have children. When they finally decide to start their families, they have already reached a low point in their ovarian supplies. On the basis of these facts, at least some women may want to make use of the possibility of retaining their fertility by freezing ovarian tissue[44,45].

HANDS OFF THE BIOLOGICAL CLOCK?

Iatrogenic loss of fertility has become a major problem for a growing number of young women because of the considerably greater likelihood of long-term survival of cancer patients (especially children)[27]. The same is true when POF is caused by a disease or other pathology. The older average age of maternity in many Western countries means that a relatively high percentage of women face premature menopause before they can have children. This fact leads to the need to re-think life plans; that, combined with physical complaints and the sense of impending aging, often leads to serious problems of adjustment[40].

All of these points support the view that an important health issue would be served by the development of techniques offering 'insurance' against the threat of both iatrogenic and pathological loss of fertility – provided we agree that (retaining) the possibility of having children that are genetically one's own is indeed an important health issue, at least for men and women of normal reproductive age[45]. (This assumption is an important pillar of accepted practices in reproductive medicine. It is, for example, the reason why ICSI is offered to couples who could also have a child through artificial insemination using donor sperm (AID), notwithstanding the smaller chances of success and the burdens and risks ICSI treatment entails for the woman, who in the majority of those cases will be normally fertile.) This viewpoint validates the first two of the three potential applications of female fertility insurance. But what of the third? In two subsequent advisory reports, the IVF-Commission of the Health Council of the Netherlands refers to 'fertility insurance for non-medical reasons' as a (morally) questionable consequence of the otherwise desirable development of the relevant technology[3,46]. A closer reading of the relevant passages in these reports reveals the striking contrast between the presentation of nonmedical applications as a problem and the complete absence of justification for that viewpoint. This contrast is echoed in a recent article in the *Netherlands Journal of Medicine*, where the authors call for ethical reflection on the conditions for introducing (experimental) cryopreservation of ovarian tissue[4]. Such reflection would require a prior normative weighing of expected moral advantages and disadvantages. One of the advantages the authors list is that when fertility is threatened by a necessary medical intervention, cryopreservation of embryos as a method of fertility insurance may be avoided. Among the disadvantages they see is the moral dilemma of 'whether retaining fertility for non-medical reasons is desirable'. Again no arguments are advanced for this judgment; the authors only hint at the possibility of important social consequences.

The clear need for providing arguments supporting the view that fertility insurance for non-medical reasons is indeed questionable will be addressed in the following sections. These arguments can be summarized under three heads: the non-medical application is undesirable because (1) it will have negative consequences for women, children, and society at large, (2) it exceeds a limit which nature herself has attached to female fertility, and (3) it makes inappropriate use of medicine and healthcare. In the following discussion of these arguments, 'fertility insurance' stands for cryopreservation of ovarian tissue as a means to ensure against natural (as opposed to iatrogenic or pathologic) loss of fertility. For the sake of argument, it is assumed that autotransplantation has been proven to be a reliable, safe method for using the frozen reserve for reproduction.

Disadvantages for women, children, and society at large?

Fertility insurance gives women the possibility of postponing childbearing, enabling them to realize many of their other life aspirations: challenging employment, a nice home, travel, and last but not least, a partner who would also qualify as a good father for their children. In the pressure cooker of these various ambitions the decision to have children is often only taken when the biological clock already points at five to twelve. How could a technology be wrong that gives women the ability to slow the ticking of that clock and bear children later on?

Consequences of late motherhood

The Health Council envisions women delaying childbearing until much later in life, 'possibly even after menopause'[46]. One reason for concern is that pregnancy at a more advanced age may entail greater risks for women. Moreover, there is concern about negative psychosocial consequences for such a child, who would be reared by older parents. These same points have been discussed in connection with the desirability of establishing an upper age limit for IVF using donor oocytes. The Health Council believes that the child's need for parental guidance up to maturity would justify an upper age limit. In addition, further research is needed to establish what

7

the age limit should be for medically assisted reproduction to be acceptable, in view of the health risks involved for the woman[46]. If these are valid
arguments for setting an upper age limit to IVF using donor oocytes[47], the
same arguments would apply to medical assistance aimed at enabling a
woman to reproduce using her own oocytes from a frozen reserve. This
presupposes, of course, that the time frame within which that reserve must
be used should be provided as part of the information preceding the decision on whether or not to have ovarian tissue cryopreserved. Presently, the
upper age limit in Dutch centers for IVF using donor oocytes is 44 at the
start of treatment. Considering the reasons for concern about late motherhood referred to earlier in this section, that seems to be a cautious position.

When considering those who would want to use fertility insurance, is it
realistic to assume that women will want to bear children at the age of 50 or
60? In view of the burdens, risks and costs of the procedure, it is much
more likely that women requesting fertility insurance will be motivated by
fear of not being able to fulfill an actual desire for motherhood than by
some hypothetical desire in a very distant future. This technology is then
most likely to be used for women in their early thirties (freezing after 35 is
probably useless) who know they want children but are not yet in a position
to have them, for example, because they have not yet found a suitable
partner[45]. Fertility insurance will give them extra time and, apart from a
hope that they can still have their own children, relief from the pressures
many women experience in that type of situation. Ten years or so extra
for late starters, what could be wrong with that?[44] The obvious answer is
medicalization!

Medicalization

Fertility insurance is a medical solution for a social problem. Currently,
society does not encourage women to bear children at that stage of their
lives when they have the best biological chance for success[48]. Regarded in
this way, fertility insurance treats symptoms that may only serve to rein-
force the underlying social problem. Pressure on women to think about
careers first and bear children later might even increase. However accurate
this objection may be in itself, it disregards the situation of individual
women who cannot step outside current social circumstances when trying
to have children in addition to whatever else they aspire to in their lives.
Furthermore, treatment of symptoms is objectionable only if it is possible
to strike at the root of the problem. It is doubtful that such is the case for
this problem. The causes of the current late average age of maternity are
too complex. The fact that many women who are at the age when they have
biologically the best chance of having children 'are still far from sure about
their partner'[49] is a cultural factor that cannot be addressed through
socio-economic measures such as day care centers and parental leave.

Moreover, if medicalization in this sense were a valid argument against fertility insurance, regular IVF would stand accused as well. Many of the women who try to give birth through IVF would not have needed medical help had they started having children ten years earlier.

Another aspect of the medicalization argument is that healthy women become dependent on medical technology for reproduction. This is not just a matter of fact, but also an emotional crutch: the hope of having a child is linked to a belief in medical technology. Whether fear of dependency in this sense is justified will hinge on how fertility insurance is presented by the profession: is it a guarantee of eternal youth or just the possibility of storing an emergency supply in case of a situation that it would be wiser not to let arise? In any case it would be unacceptable to give false hopes, which can be avoided by providing adequate information as part of the counseling that precedes a woman's decision, that is informing her about what is realistically possible after thawing of the tissue.

Against nature?

Is what makes fertility insurance undesirable the fact that it is intended as a means of going beyond a limit to the human condition set by nature herself? This cannot mean that human beings must not interfere with natural processes (that would amount to an absurd and untenable argument). Medicine, for example, constantly interferes with nature, and we are happy it does. At first sight a more plausible version of the argument from nature was advanced by the Dutch ethicist H Zwart, who called for differentiation between interventions that respect the inherent directedness of the processes of life and those that do not[50]. Prescribing antibiotics to fight a bacterial infection is consistent with the tendency towards recovery of health inherent in nature. By contrast, there is no such consistency with nature if ART is used to help postmenopausal women who have lost their fertility at a normal age. Medicine then acts against nature. But does this also necessarily make such actions undesirable (and if so, why)?[47] The natural loss of ovarian function not only leads to infertility but also changes a woman's hormonal balance. If the gametogenic function of the ovary should not be replaced because it would be against nature, would not the same argument be valid for hormonal supplements that treat complaints resulting from the loss of the steroidogenic function?[51] Conversely, if this application is valid as an acceptable form of 'not respecting' the natural limit of ovarian aging, why would the same not hold for the previous one? According to Gosden, the early fertility loss of modern women, in view of their life expectancy, amounts to a 'biological inequity', from which the technology he has developed may help them escape[44]. Why should they submit to the dictates of nature?

The main objection to the naturalness argument is that it is we who interpret nature's 'intent'. It is not nature setting limits, but we are the ones doing so, and subsequently what we regard as acceptable we call 'natural' and the rest 'unnatural' or 'perverse'[52]. There is nothing wrong with our doing this so long as we do not present these arguments as reasons for the acceptability or unacceptability of certain practices or actions.

Inappropriate use of medicine and healthcare?

H. M. Kuitert (one of the founding fathers of medical ethics in the Netherlands) states that the goal of medicine is to help people escape the evils of disease, physical handicaps and premature death[53]. In his view, doctors should refrain from interventions that are not included in one of these categories because they would be inappropriate medicine. His concern is that if medicine is not restricted to the domains of curing and healing, doctors become authorities beyond their realm of competence, where they cannot tell if their interventions are beneficial or not. The boundary which Kuitert and other authors point at here is understood as inherent in the profession of medicine itself, regarded as a moral practice with a clearly-defined goal. In this connection, reference is often made to 'the internal morality of medicine'[54].

Between essentialism and positivism

Fertility insurance where no disease is present (such as cases of threatening iatrogenic or pathologic fertility loss) falls outside the scope of curing and healing. Does this mean that gynecologists should not accede to requests for this type of intervention? G. M. de Wert believes that definitions of the goal of medicine, such as the one given by Kuitert, may be helpful as a description of what is traditionally regarded as the core of medicine, but without providing a sharp delineation of what is appropriate medicine and what is not[55]. Beyond that core, there is a periphery of activities not directly related to the primary goal of curing and healing; many of these peripheral activities have acquired a place within the field of medicine. Two examples are plastic surgery for cosmetic reasons ('facelifts') and sterilization in the context of family planning. As de Wert remarks, it would be difficult to maintain that doctors performing such activities are engaging in improper behavior because they do not fit in the traditional view of medicine's mission. He suspects the argument is guilty of 'medico-moral essentialism'.

Does this line of reasoning, however, go one step too far, ending up in 'medico-moral positivism' (a variation of de Wert's own terminology)? That would be true if he intends the difference between core and periphery to be regarded as important solely for historical or descriptive reasons, but having no normative association. Between the extremes of essentialism (goal and limits as laid down once and for all in the 'essence' of medicine) and positivism (medicine as the mere application of medical technology), a third possibility is that even though medicine has no distinctive boundaries (if only because concepts such as disease and health defy unambiguous definition), there is still a normative stratification. Some things doctors do (at the core) are more legitimately a part of medicine than are other activities (at the periphery), and the more peripheral activities require justification in how they relate to the core[54].

Fertility insurance as enhancement

In any event fertility insurance cannot be regarded as treatment of disease or handicap. Rather, the intervention falls in the category of 'enhancements', defined by Juengst as 'interventions aimed at healthy systems and normal traits'[56]. To speak of an enhancement in this context (rather than a mutilating intervention), we must regard the frozen tissue as a disconnected extension of the woman's follicular reserve still present *in vivo*. That does not seem inappropriate, since the woman herself will also look at it that way, and because the tissue is intended to be re-inserted in her body in due course. The measure extends the woman's reproductive lifespan, thus giving her a better chance to fulfill her desire for motherhood in addition to achieving other aims. The intervention therefore leads to a (subjective) enhancement of a normal physical condition, just as is the case in cosmetic surgery aimed at correcting the outward signs of aging, or in pharmaco logical interventions aimed at enhancing the cognitive abilities of people having normal intellectual capabilities. As a form of enhancement, however, fertility insurance seems to fall in the category of interventions that may be outside the sphere of medicine.

Let us examine whether this is consistent with the situation in which a woman desiring to have children can no longer become pregnant herself but, having preserved some ovarian tissue, requests medical help to use that tissue for reproductive purposes. Assume that this woman is in her early forties and that she hopes that the autotransplant procedures will give her additional years to become pregnant with her own oocytes, either naturally or, should that prove impossible, through IVF. Would her request be rejected as an inappropriate use of medicine? That position would be difficult to defend, given the fact that women above the age of 40 are still accepted for IVF using donor oocytes. It would be strange if medical assistance for this woman were to be limited to reproduction using someone else's oocytes but not her own. Nor is it a valid argument that she waited too long to bear children. Her age does not change her condition; moreover, the same is true of many women who depend on IVF (with or without donor oocytes) for the fulfillment of their desire for children.

11

Finally, 'it's your own fault' is not viewed as an acceptable criterion for granting or withholding medical help in other areas of medicine[47].

How, then, is the relationship between storage (enhancement) and use of the reserve (treatment) to be seen? How can the one be outside the scope of medicine while the other clearly falls within it? Juengst points to the fact that if the distinction between treatment and enhancement is used to delineate between what legitimately belongs to medicine and what does not, a problem arises with the notion of prevention. Measures aimed at preventing disease in individuals are always regarded as a part of medicine, meaning that they fall within 'the treatment side of the enhancement boundary'[56]. But some of those measures can be conceived as enhancements aimed at preventing future health problems. An example is enhancement of the immune system through vaccination against infectious diseases. Can fertility insurance also be regarded as a form of 'preventive enhancement'? After all, the measure is intended to prevent a health problem (infertility, or at least its consequence: involuntary childlessness) in women who want children but are not yet in a position to bear them.

Fertility insurance as prevention

Whether prevention is a useful concept here depends on the appropriateness of calling future infertility a health problem. Does not the essentially natural character of that condition exclude the possibility that it is a health problem? In the course of the debate about whether postmenopausal women should be admitted to IVF using donor oocytes, the Canadian Royal Commission took a clear stance when they stated, 'because it is normal for women to be infertile at this age, there is no medical justification for the practice'[57]. This was also the position of the French legislature, which stipulated that assisted reproduction is only for women 'en âge de procréer' (who are in their childbearing years)[58]. There is another side to this debate, however. In the Netherlands, official support for an opposite view was expressed in reports by commissions of both the Royal Netherlands Medical Association (KNMG) and the Health Council. They argued that in the field of reproductive medicine it is not possible without inconsistency to differentiate between natural and non-natural causes of infertility[46,59]. Both Dutch reports urged that an upper age limit for IVF using donor oocytes be implemented, but only because of possible health risks of pregnancy for older women (which should be investigated further) and possible negative psycho-social consequences for the child to be. Wherever that limit may be set, the essential point is that the natural infertility of postmenopausal women is not seen as standing in the way of medically assisted reproduction. If this means that infertility, in so far as it leads to unwanted childlessness, is as such a health problem, whatever its natural or non-natural causes, it is also possible to view fertility insurance as a preventive measure. Timely freezing of ovarian tissue could help avoid the health problem of having to remain involuntarily childless.

However, that conclusion, and the reasoning on which it rests, tend to obscure the distinction between a health problem and an unwanted condition. When that distinction loses definition, the notion of fertility insurance as a form of prevention loses its rationale: it becomes possible to claim a legitimate place within medicine for every intervention that leads to an enhancement of the quality of life. If this is an unacceptable consequence, we may consider that sufficient reason to retain the Canadian Royal Commission's position that natural infertility, however unwanted, cannot be a health problem. (Whether that position can be maintained in the long run remains to be seen. What would be the implications for the concept of 'natural infertility' if science were to yield a simple pill that could retard or temporarily stop the follicular depletion process in the ovaries?[60] If such a technology made it possible to extend the age at which women reach menopause, would the 'âge de procréer' be similarly extended?) But is the notion of natural infertility necessary here? Only in so far as women want to have the option of bearing children after menopause. If, however, the earlier assumption is correct, fertility insurance is really a matter of providing additional time for late starters. This means that the situation is not so much natural infertility, but rather the preceding condition of progressive fertility loss. It is not possible to delineate in the decade preceding menopause exactly where fertility stops and infertility begins. Because of their reduced fertility and poor chances of success, as a rule women over 40 will no longer have an indication for regular IVF. All the same, their unwanted childlessness is regarded as a health problem constituting an indication for treatment using donor oocytes. Even though they are at the edge of their childbearing years, these women are still eligible for assisted reproduction. As argued above, it would be strange if that assistance were to exclude reproduction using their own frozen oocytes.

What is considered is not cryopreservation of ovarian tissue intended for reproductive use after menopause. It remains questionable whether that is a medical issue. Here it is a matter of cryopreservation of ovarian tissue intended for use in that twilight period between fertile and infertile years. The notion of fertility insurance as a form of prevention seems defensible if it is an issue of enabling women who are trapped in time to extend by a number of years the period in which they may have children using their own oocytes. In any event, this means that the enhancement character of the measure is not as such a reason to regard the granting of a cryopreservation request as an inappropriate use of medicine.

'First do no harm'

Before freezing the tissue, it needs harvesting. Does the invasive nature of the (usually) necessary oophorectomy or biopsy provide a sufficient reason for doctors to refrain from the intervention? Biopsy is used for harvesting a limited amount of tissue, as opposed to complete removal of one or both ovaries. Although it entails a less extensive operation, the laparoscopic procedure is usually performed under general anesthesia and cannot be regarded as an intervention of negligible risk[61]. Those who believe that a doctor should not subject a patient (not even at her own request) to burdensome and risky interventions without a clear medical necessity, would have to conclude that harvesting ovarian tissue as infertility insurance for non-medical reasons cannot be justified. The intervention would amount to a violation of the medical–ethical principle 'first do no harm' (*primum non nocere*). All the same, this reason need not rule out fertility insurance completely. Gosden points to the fact that patients undergoing an abdominal operation or Caesarean section could have ovarian tissue frozen without the need for a separate operation[44]. As he says, it might also be possible to freeze immature oocytes obtained with minimal risk from unstimulated ovaries through vaginal puncture. However, since no more than five or ten such oocytes can be harvested per cycle, the build-up of a useful reserve would require a greater number of punctures, thereby increasing the total burden involved for the woman.

If this position (no exposure to more than negligible burdens or risks without clear medical need) is viewed as too restrictive (especially given the preventive element discussed above), the issue becomes under which conditions would the intervention be acceptable. The American ethicist J.A. Robertson argues that it would depend on balancing the benefits fertility insurance may provide for the woman in question against the possible risks attendant on the intervention[62]. This means, he says, that oophorectomy (excision of a complete ovary) can only be justified in exceptional cases, namely if the woman knows 'to a high degree of certainty' that she will not reproduce in her fertile years. If a less invasive biopsy is performed, the risk-to-benefit ratio can be expected to be more favorable, making that procedure more easily justified[63].

Which situations would satisfy Robertson's requirement of a high degree of certainty about delayed childbearing? One of these could be a female prisoner foreseeing that after long-term detention she would no longer be able to become pregnant using her own oocytes[64]. Or perhaps a female linguist without a partner working in the jungle of New Guinea on a project codifying the language of an isolated Papuan tribe: she does not want to abandon her commitment to that long-term project and the people there because of the ticking of her biological clock. In such cases there is an objective (external or internal) impediment that works against timely reproduction. Robertson's criterion seems to exclude women who are

'only' concerned that they will not be able to have children befor
out of oocytes. In their case there is no 'high degree of certainty'
cannot reproduce before it is too late, but only a growing uncerta
is felt more acutely with each passing year. But does this fact le:
benefit of fertility insurance for these women? Any woman in her ea
ties who wants children but has not yet found the partner with whom to fulfill that desire has no sure knowledge as to whether cryopreservation of her
ovarian tissue may turn out to have been unnecessary. Nor can her gynecologist tell her. If she meets 'Mr Right' quickly, they will not have to use
the frozen tissue, but if he keeps her waiting for another ten years, that
reserve may mean the difference between having (her own) children or
not, just as it would for the prisoner or the linguist. Moreover, the benefit
fertility insurance may have for the woman will depend on individual factors, such as the intensity of her desire for children and the impact of having more time for fulfilling various ambitions (including motherhood) may
have on the quality of her life. Because such considerations have a strong
personal character, assessment of the risk-to-benefit ratio in specific cases
will require individual counseling[65].

When assessing this ratio there is another factor to be considered. Harvesting ovarian tissue entails a reduction of the follicular reserve still present *in vivo*. Depending on the quantity of harvested tissue, this may mean
that natural loss of fertility sets in earlier than would otherwise have been
the case[23]. It is not inconceivable that the intervention (especially
oophorectomy) may well preclude the possibility of having a child before
infertility sets in, should circumstances turn out to be favorable for childbearing after all. Considering the principle of 'first do no harm' would
such an intervention ever be justifiable? It is difficult to imagine, even
admitting exceptional cases that fit Robertson's 'high degree of certainty'
criterion. If there is no medical necessity for the intervention, it can only be
justifiable to harvest (through biopsy) so much ovarian tissue as can be rec-
onciled with the requirement that the natural reproductive potential of the
woman should not be (or only barely be) affected by the procedure. In this
respect it makes no difference if the harvesting intervention would require
a separate operation.

Inappropriate use of healthcare funding?

A final objection is that, in countries with collective funding of ART, fertility insurance would encroach on the means available for healthcare, thus
violating the principle of justice. Here again, we should differentiate
between harvesting and storage of ovarian tissue on the one hand, and
making the oocytes it contains available for reproductive use on the other.
In so far as medically assisted use of the frozen reserve (autotransplantation with or without subsequent IVF treatment) may be requested in that

15

twilight period between fertile and infertile years, it seems difficult to argue that collective funding of the necessary procedures would be inappropriate. After all, the woman would otherwise still be eligible to undergo IVF using donor oocytes as a collectively funded healthcare provision. For harvesting and storage, however, collective funding would seem indefensible since there is no health problem at the time of the request. The fact that storage is intended to prevent a possible health problem in the future does not enter into consideration. Not all conceivable preventive measures need to be provided as a part of healthcare. The cost of obtaining, freezing and preserving the tissue would therefore have to be borne by the woman wishing the procedure, possibly through supplementary insurance. It should be noted that for exceptional cases, in which a complication of the harvesting procedure may necessitate medical treatment, the collective healthcare system will be called upon. It would be difficult to see this as a serious objection to making fertility insurance an available option.

CONCLUSION

The argument that fertility insurance for healthy women is undesirable cannot be convincingly based on 'medicalization', 'respect for nature' or the need to guard the boundaries of medicine and healthcare. Nor are there grounds for maintaining that this application would constitute a moral dilemma with regard to the desirable development of relevant techniques for helping women who, as a consequence of medical treatment or disease, face the threat of premature menopause. For women who feel trapped by time, freezing of ovarian tissue may mean the difference between having or not having children that are genetically their own. If 'preventive enhancement' is not a mistaken qualification, there may even be reason to regard the availability of that option (extra time for late starters) as desirable from a health perspective, in addition to measures aimed at stimulating women to start having children earlier in their lives.

How does this conclusion affect the present situation in which it is possible to freeze ovarian tissue, but without any certainty that it will be possible to use that reserve for future reproduction? Freezing the tissue now is performed to allow for using it then. What is still uncertain now (the possibility of recovery of fertility after autotransplantation) may be proven. In anticipation of scientific developments, cryopreservation of ovarian tissue is already being carried out on cancer patients. Should that option also be offered to healthy women who fear they may not be able to become mothers? Why not cryopreserve some of their tissue as well, thus allowing them to profit from future scientific research? One good argument for not yet engaging in this intervention is that harvesting of ovarian tissue implies a reduction of the follicular reserve present *in vivo*. As long as the results of the procedure are uncertain, it cannot be excluded that the intervention would on balance reduce rather than enhance reproductive ability. One of the pioneers of research in this field, the Frenchman Y. Aubard, believes that indications for experimental cryopreservation should, for the time being, be limited to cases in which the woman has 'nothing to lose'[20]. This includes women undergoing medical treatment that will either result in menopause or else lead to a dramatic reduction of their follicular reserve[23]. This applies to specific cancer treatments such as total body irradiation, high-dose alkylating chemotherapy, combined abdominal radiotherapy and chemotherapy. Women with an increased risk of pathologic fertility loss do not satisfy Aubard's criterion, as the precise risk of ovarian failure cannot be known in individual cases. For those women, experimental cryopreservation could mean losing a last opportunity for spontaneous conception without any assurance of future benefit. For the present, the 'nothing to lose' criterion also excludes women desiring insurance against natural loss of fertility. As long as it remains uncertain that insurance will provide added benefit, they risk ending up with fewer rather than more fertile years[23].

REFERENCES

1. Silber SJ. *How to Get Pregnant With the New Technology*, updated and revised edition. New York: Warner Books, 1998
2. The Genetics and IVF Institute. *Ovary Cryopreservation (Ovarian Freezing, Egg Banking)*. http://www.givf.com/ovary.cfm
3. Health Council of the Netherlands. Committee on *In vitro* fertilization. *IVF-related Research*. Rijswijk, 1998; publ. nr 1998/08E
4. Hilhorst JA, Braat DDM, Goverde HJM, Ten Have HAMJ. Cryopreservatie van ovariumweefsel; ethische bezinning nu opportuun [in Dutch]. *Ned Tijds Geneesk* 2000;144:695–8
5. Picton HM, Kim SS, Gosden RG. Cryopreservation of gonadal tissue and cells. *Br Med Bull* 2000;56:603–15
6. Donnez J, Godin PA, Qu J, *et al*. Gonadal cryopreservation in the young patient with gynaecological malignancy. *Curr Opin Obstet Gynecol* 2000;12:1–9
7. Atkinson HG, Apperley JF, Goldman JM, *et al*. Successful pregnancy after allogeneic bone marrow transplantation for chronic myeloid leukaemia. *Lancet* 1994;344:199
8. Braat DDM, Schattenberg AVMB. Kan een vrouw na stamceltransplantatie nog zwanger worden? [in Dutch] *Ned Tijds Geneesk* 2000;144:689–91
9. Oktay K, Newton H, Aubard Y, *et al*. Cryopreservation of immature human oocytes and ovarian tissue: an emerging technology? *Fertil Steril* 1998;69:1–7
10. Porcu E. Freezing of oocytes. *Curr Opin Obstet Gynecol* 1999;11:297–300
11. Smitz J, Cortvrindt R. Oocyte in-vitro maturation and follicle culture: current clinical achievements and future directions. *Hum Reprod* 1999;14:145–61
12. Newton H, Aubard Y, Rutherford A, *et al*. Low temperature storage and grafting of human ovarian tissue. *Hum Reprod* 1996;11:1487–91

13.   Nugent D, Meirow D, Brook PF, *et al*. Transplantation in reproductive medicine: previous experience, present knowledge and future prospects. *Hum Reprod Update* 1997;3:267–80
14.   Kim SS, Battaglia DE, Soules MR. The future of human ovarian cryopreservation and transplantation: fertility and beyond. *Fertil Steril* 2001;75:1049–56
15.   Oktay K, Karlikaya GG, Aydin BA. Ovarian cryotransplantation and transplantation: basic aspects. *Mol Cell Endocrinol* 2000;169:105–8
16.   Aubard Y, Newton H, Scheffer G, *et al*. Conservation of the follicular population in irradiated rats by the cryopreservation and orthotopic autografting of ovarian tissue. *Eur J Obstet Gynecol Reprod Biol* 1998;79:83–7
17.   Shaw JM, Cox SL, Trounson AO, *et al*. Evaluation of the long-term function of cryopreserved ovarian grafts in the mouse, implications for human applications. *Mol Cell Endocrinol* 2000;161:103–10
18.   Gosden RG, Baird DT, Wade JC, *et al*. Restoration of fertility to oophorectomized sheep by ovarian autografts stored at –196 degrees C. *Hum Reprod* 1994;9:597–603
19.   Baird DT, Webb R, Campbell BK, *et al*. Long-term ovarian function in sheep after ovariectomy and transplantation of autografts stored at –196°C. *Endocrinology* 1999;140:462–70
20.   Aubard Y. Ovarian tissue graft: from animal experiment to practice in the human. *Eur J Obstet Gynecol* 1999;86:1–3
21.   Linch DC, Gosden RG, Tulandi T, Tan SL, Hancock SL. Hodgkin's lymphoma: choice of therapy and late complications. *Hematology* (Am Soc Hematol Educ Program) 2001;1:205–21
22.   Donnez J, Bassil S. Indications for cryopreservation of ovarian tissue. *Hum Reprod Update* 1998;4:248–59
23.   Aubard Y, Piver P, Teisseir MP. Indications de la cryopréservation du tissu ovarien. *La Presse Médicale* 2000;29:960–4
24.   Oktay K, Karlikaya G. Ovarian function after transplantation of frozen, banked autologous ovarian tissue. *N Engl J Med* 2000;342:1919
25.   Radford JA, Lieberman BA, Brison DR, *et al*. Orthotopic reimplantation of cryopreserved ovarian cortical strips after high-dose chemotherapy for Hodgkin's lymphoma. *Lancet* 2001;357:1172–5
26.   Shaw JM, Bowles J, Koopman P, *et al*. Fresh and cryopreserved ovarian tissue samples from donors with lymphoma transmit the cancer to graft recipients. *Hum Reprod* 1996;11:1668–73
27.   Gosden RG. Trade-offs in cancer and reproduction. *Hum Reprod Update* 2001;7:360–2
28.   Meirow D. Ovarian tissue banking in patients with Hodgkin's disease: is it safe? *Fertil Steril* 1998;69:996–8
29.   Meirow D. Reproduction post-chemotherapy in young cancer patients. *Mol Cell Endocrinol* 2000;169:123–31
30.   Gosden RG, Rutherford AJ, Norfolk DR. Ovarian banking for cancer patients. Transmission of malignant cells in ovarian grafts. *Hum Reprod* 1997;12:403
31.   Health Council of the Netherlands. Committee on xenotransplantation. *Xenotransplantation*. Rijswijk, 1998; publicatie nr 1998/01E

32. Oktay K, Nugent D, Newton H, *et al*. Isolation and characterization of primordial follicles from fresh and cryopreserved human ovarian tissue. *Fertil Steril* 1997;67:481–6

33. Eppig JJ, O'Brien MJ. Development *in vitro* of mouse oocytes from primordial follicles. *Biol Reprod* 1996;54:197–207

34. Heineman MJ. Het invriezen van ovaria. Optie voor vrouwen die hun vruchtbaarheid verliezen als gevolg van een oncologische behandeling? *Tijdschrift Kanker* 1998;22:32–4

35. Tinga DJ, Dolsma WV, Tamminga RYJ, *et al*. Behoud van de ovariële functie bij 2 jonge vrouwen met de ziekte van Hodgkin, door laparoscopische transpositie van de ovaria voorafgaand aan abdominale bestraling. *Ned Tijds Geneesk* 1999;143:308–12

36. Meirow D. Ovarian injury and modern options to preserve fertility in female cancer patients treated with high dose radio-chemotherapy for hemato-oncological neoplasias and other cancers. *Leuk Lymph* 1999;33:65–76

37. de Sutter P. Gender reassignment and assisted reproduction. Present and future reproductive options for transsexual people. *Hum Reprod* 2001;16: 612–14

38. van Kasteren YM, Schoemaker J. Premature ovarian failure: a systematic review of therapeutic interventions to restore ovarian function and achieve pregnancy. *Hum Reprod Update* 1999;5:483–92

39. Laml T, Schulz-Lobmeyr I, Obruca A, *et al*. Premature ovarian failure: etiology and prospects. *Gynecol Endocrinol* 2000;14:292–302

40. van Kasteren YM. Prematuur ovarieel falen. *Ned Tijds Geneesk* 2000;144: 2142–6

41. Schuiling GA. Early menopause? *J Psychosom Obstet Gynecol* 2001;22:123–6

42. Centraal Bureau voor de Statistiek. *Vademecum Gezondheidsstatistiek Nederland 2000*. Voorburg/Heerlen/Den Haag, 2000

43. Bonsel GJ, van der Maas PJ. *Aan de wieg van de toekomst. Scenario's voor de zorg rond de menselijke voortplanting 1995–2010*. Houten/Diegem: Bohn Stafleu Van Loghum, 1994

44. Gosden R, Tan SL, Oktay K. Oocytes for late starters and posterity: are we on to something good or bad? *Fertil Steril* 2000;74:1057–8

45. de Wert GMWR, de Beaufort ID. Cryopreservatie van ovariumweefsel ter discussie. *Ned Tijds Geneesk* 2000;144:692–4

46. Health Council of the Netherlands. Committee on *in vitro* fertilization. *In Vitro Fertilization (IVF)*. Rijswijk, 1997; publ.nr 1997/03E

47. de Wert GMWR. The post-menopause: playground for reproductive technology? Some ethical reflections. In: Harris J, Holm S, eds. *The Future of Human Reproduction. Ethics, Choice, and Regulation*. Oxford: Clarendon Press, 1998:221–37

48. Emancipatieraad. *Het late ouderschap: over uitstel en afstel. Advies maatschappelijke consequenties uitgesteld ouderschap*. Den Haag: Emancipatieraad, 1996

49. Becker H (Professor of Sociology). *Algemeen Dagblad*, 07-08-01

50. Zwart H. *De natuur als argument in de ethiek*. Pre-advies Ned Vereniging Bioethiek. Utrecht: NVBe, 1995

51. Rieger D. Gamete donation: an opinion on the recommendations of the Royal Commission on New Reproductive Technologies. *Can Med Assoc J* 1994;151:1433–5

52. van Willigenburg T. *Ethiek: denken tegen het vooroordeel. Over verborgen moralismen en rationaliteit.* Utrecht: Stichting Socrates, 1997

53. Kuitert HM. *Mag alles wat kan? Ethiek en medisch handelen.* Baarn: Ten Have, 1989

54. Miller FG, Brody H, Chung KC. Cosmetic surgery and the internal morality of medicine. *Cambr Q Healthcare Eth* 2000;9:353–64

55. de Wert GMWR. *Met het oog op de toekomst. Voortplantingstechnologie, erfelijkheidsonderzoek en ethiek.* Amsterdam: Thela Thesis, 1999

56. Juengst ET. What does *enhancement* mean? In: Parens E, ed. *Enhancing Human Traits: Ethical and Social Implications.* Washington DC: Georgetown University Press, 1998:29–47

57. Royal Commission on New Reproductive Technologies. *Proceed with Care. Final Report of the Royal Commission on New Reproductive Technologies.* Ottawa, 1993

58. Loi no 94-654 du 29 juillet 1994 relative au don et à l'utilisation des éléments et produits du corps humain, à l'assistance médicale à la procréation et au diagnostic prénatal. *J Officiel* 1994;126

59. KNMG, commissie medische ethiek. IVF op latere leeftijd. *Medisch Contact* 1996;51:620–7

60. Ainsworth C. Fertility in the freezer. Can we help women to keep their eggs forever? *New Sci* 30-06-2001:38–43

61. Grundy R, Larcher V, Gosden RG, *et al.* Fertility preservation for children treated for cancer (2): ethics of consent for gamete storage and experimentation. *Arch Dis Child* 2001;84:360–2

62. Robertson JA. Ethical issues in ovarian transplantation and donation (editorial). *Fertil Steril* 2000;74:443–6

63. Robertson JA. Author's reply. *Fertil Steril* 2000;74:1057–8

64. Lee RG, Morgan D. *Human Fertilisation & Embryology. Regulating the Reproductive Revolution.* London: Blackstone, 2001

65. Veatch RM. Doctor does not know best: why in the new century physicians must stop trying to benefit patients. *J Med Philos.* 2000;25:701–21

2

Attempts to preserve the reproductive capability of minors with cancer: who should give consent?

F. Shenfield, M. C. Davies and H. A. Spoudeas

THE NEW DILEMMA FACING REPRODUCTIVE SPECIALISTS

It behoves all working in the reproductive arena to pause and consider a new moral dilemma, that is whether to attempt to preserve the reproductive potential of cancer sufferers, particularly of children and adolescents. Of the latter 70% survive to face an uncertain future with significant psychologic and medical morbidity. The reproductive field is especially fraught with psychosocial issues. Adolescents are usually concerned with potential potency rather than fertility, while legal and ethical dilemmas abound in the area of informed consent, particularly because it is a quality rather than quantity of life issue. As such, ensuring access to the 'child's voice' is a crucial factor in acting together in their best interest[1], thus balancing a respect for their autonomy with parental and medical opinions. It may be argued that physicians familiar with obtaining informed consent in adults with reproductive failure are not best placed or trained to talk to children. Pediatricians, and child mental health professionals, may be better at the latter and are bound by their code of practice to act in the child's best interests[2], but may lack knowledge and experience in the legal and medical aspects of assisted reproductive technology (ART). It is therefore of vital importance to begin an open dialog between these multidisciplinary groups, in order to resolve this difficult and potentially highly contentious area.

THE FACTS

What is known about gonadotoxicity?

The facts are stark: one in 650 children will develop cancer by the age of 16, of whom some 70% will be cured; 5–10% of these long-term survivors will develop a second primary tumor[3]. This means that 1 in 1000 young adults (aged 20–30 years) in the UK today has survived childhood cancer[4], which is further estimated to increase to 1 in 250 in the next decade as survival is further prolonged.

Approximately 10–15% of young survivors have received intensive treatment carrying a substantial (> 80%) risk to their fertility[5]. The risk certainty depends on the total cumulative dose of gonadotoxic chemotherapeutic agents or radiation, the underlying tumor, its position relative to the reproductive organs and the age and sex of the child, but even in the most gonadotoxic regimens it is nearer 95% than 100%[6,7]. Males are particularly affected by alkylating agents and testicular irradiation[8], while females who have radiation therapy to the abdomen have decreased fertility and an increased risk of adverse pregnancy outcome owing to uterine dysfunction, with a potential requirement to consider surrogacy because of irradiation-induced uterine fibrosis[9,10].

Until the advent of IVF and related techniques the only potential 'insurance strategy' against possible infertility was – and this for the postpubertal, intellectually competent male child only – cryopreservation of gametes prior to treatment. Egg donation, intracytoplasmic sperm injection (ICSI) with ejaculated or testicular gametes, oocyte cryopreservation and now experimental gonadal tissue freezing (perhaps even human reproductive cloning), have since offered new hope to cancer patients. Indeed, the first successful follicular development in autografted previously cryopreserved ovarian tissue[11] and the restoration of the menstrual cycle after orthotopic autotransplantation of cryopreserved ovarian cortical strips in a young woman after a sterilizing dose of chemotherapy[12] have, despite premature failure rate and a requirement for ongoing stimulation, attracted intense media interest and made specialists and patients aware of new technologies.

MALE AND FEMALE DIFFERENCES

There is an inherent inequality between males and females in the reproductive field, which is, of course a joint project between the two genders and requires the previous existence of a partnership and sexual relationship, something that is less common in cancer survivors[13].

Male gametes

Obtaining and ensuring treatment with cryopreserved sperm is easy and routine if the male is adult, healthy, fully virilized and sexually active. If the sperm is of good enough quality it can be used in straightforward insemination, but if the sperm is of poor quality, conception involves the patient's partner being prepared to undergo stimulated cycles towards IVF or IVF/ ICSI, techniques regulated in the UK under the Human Fertilisation and

Embryology Act 1990[14]. Unfortunately, sperm quality may well be reduced in patients with malignancy, particularly lymphoma or testicular teratoma[15,16], while in the younger peripubertal patient, there may be inadequate virilization, poor health, cultural or emotional reasons for being unable to produce an adequate specimen. Although time and disease remission may enhance co-operative understanding and success, it is unclear what effects, if any, ongoing chemotherapy may have on existing sperm, and storage is usually attempted prior to treatment.

In the developing male, primary spermatocytes appear at the beginning of puberty; the presence of sperm in the urine (spermaturia) gives an indicator of the potential likelihood of spermatogenesis some 6 months previously, the latter requiring adequate intratesticular testosterone. However, the ability to masturbate and the likely success of sperm storage may require an even higher level of testosterone such as might only be possible in pubertal stage 3/4. Spermarche, defined by the appearance of spermaturia, occurs at a median age of 13 years but with a wide range (range 9–16)[17], and children as young as 11 years have successfully banked sperm although the success rate in our unit has been only 50% at this age (Bahadur, personal communication). Sperm may be present even when there is little or no pubic hair with testicular volumes of just 4 ml[18]. More research is needed to correlate the ability to store sperm with Tanner classification of pubertal stage. In 274 sperm analyses from 134 prepubertal boys, azoospermia dominates from the first ejaculation to 5/12, oligospermia from 6/12 to 11/12, asthenospermia from 12 to 20/12 and normospermia is only present after 21 months. Although testicular tissue freezing may prove a future option for young boys who do not produce sperm in their ejaculate, it is entirely unproven and carries a significant risk of harm[19]. Finally there is always the possibility of spontaneous recovery, which is irradiation dose- and fractionation-dependent[8] and increases with time[20], even after chemotherapy. Given the potential of ICSI where even men with azoospermia have fathered children[21], this possibility needs to be given greater weight than hitherto.

Female gametes

The older the female, the more likely the same gonadotoxic insult will destroy rather than reduce ovarian reserve, as the fixed ovarian pool decreases with age[22]. Thus it is the youngest (infant) female patients receiving the most gonadotoxic therapies who are the ones in whom experimental ovarian tissue cryopreservation protection strategies are most indicated and theoretically most likely to work. However, paradoxically these children are also most likely to be the sickest, with the greatest risk of disease-related death (from transplants, pelvic bone tumors), and in whom the procedures may be technically hazardous or difficult; in addition they also are likely to retain a potential window of fertility, despite an early menopause[23].

For the postpubertal female, the option of harvesting mature oocytes has recently become available, but requires a stimulated cycle and vaginal or laparoscopic collection. The alternative, for both the pre- and postpubertal child, is to obtain gonadal tissue, which may require a gonadectomy. In a large French survey the complication rate of diagnostic laparoscopy was estimated at 1.84 per 1000 procedures, and the overall complication rate for both diagnostic and operative laparoscopy was 4.64 per 1000[24]. These would be higher in a child because of the potential requirement for laparotomy owing to the technical difficulties of laparoscopy in young children, and an increased risk of infection and bleeding, especially in hematological and/or pelvic malignancies.

The technical difficulties concerning the cryopreservation of immature and mature oocytes have stimulated the development of the storage of ovarian tissue. Indeed, cryopreservation of metaphase II oocytes had very poor results[25], although recent progress[26] means a possible 5% success rate, arguably enough to justify oocyte freezing. There is also research using *in vitro* maturation (IVM) of immature oocytes collected in unstimulated cycles[27]. Another alternative is the very topical freezing of ovarian tissue, with the possibility of later autografting when the young woman has recovered and wishes to procreate. However, there is at least a theoretical risk of transmitting malignant cells in autografted slices of ovaries[28], although a recent report is reassuring, at least when samples are taken in disease remission[29].

Ovarian tissue autografts remain unproven with unknown risks. In the child these risks may be increased. The risks have to be balanced with the outlook of doing nothing and with the 30% success of oocyte donation (OD)[30]. In OD the gestating component of gravidity often psychologically repairs and counterbalances the lack of genetic input for the female patient[31].

AN UNKNOWN FUTURE

Thus we address a problem which can only loom larger, as a result of both the improved survival from childhood cancer and the increased interest (largely from profit-making fertility centers) to harvest and manipulate gonadal tissue for the purpose of future reproduction. As adults and physicians we are making two assumptions: first that all cancer survivors wish to have children and will form stable partnerships, and second that, without our intervention, the case for fertility is otherwise hopeless and the procedure itself is relatively harmless and virtually proven. Is this actually the case?

First, the evidence suggests that cancer survivors do not have children for many reasons, including failure to form sexual partnerships and fear of relapse and early death as well as infertility[13]. Second, even in the most gonadotoxic transplant regimens, there is a 2–5% spontaneous delivery rate[6] of healthy children which may increase as survival is further prolonged. Do we have the evidence that we can improve on these spontaneous pregnancy rates without inducing 'more than negligible harm'? This is the criterion used if some of the techniques, especially ovarian tissue cryopreservation, are considered research rather than therapy[32]. The harm may be both physical (including harming the existing 5% chance of spontaneous fertility) and psychological (including falsely raising hopes), and its assessment should include both the patient and his/her future offspring. Can we reassure each potential parent that current cryopreservation and micromanipulation techniques to generate gametes or autografts are safe to both the parent and the genetic progeny? This complexity entails various specific ethical issues in this field, further magnified by legal issues of competence in children.

Legal issues concerning consent by incompetent minors

The first concern is of a psychological nature. While the burden of the disease process is often reflected in the compliance problems that many children and adolescents experience, children often assume that offers are prescriptive, and may view the option of storing gametes or gonadal tissue as a 'must' rather than a 'may'. This problem should be elicited during the process of obtaining informed consent. In the legal sense, of course, we are accustomed in the UK to differentiating between the obligatory 'must' of legislation, and the 'should' of codes of practice from Royal Colleges or other professional/regulatory bodies, which sometimes may be cited in court as references of good practice and treated as normative. In the ethical sense, in spite of the ethical dimension of the legal professional duty of care (with both beneficent and non-maleficent intent) this particular field is even more fraught than others with a possible conflict of interests. This may happen while weighing these duties, the future benefits of research and the need to respect the autonomy of the child, and also considering the wishes of his/her parents. Legally this autonomy is translated into giving consent and applying the test of what is in the best interests of the child.

A minor's consent to treatment

In the UK a child of 16 has the right to give consent to medical treatment[33]. Legal problems of consent for those under 16 fall within the remit of the Gillick case and the notion of Gillick competence, which made legal precedent[34]. This case challenged the concept that a doctor could pre-scribe treatment (in this case contraception) to an underage girl without her parents' knowledge. The appeal at the House of Lords clearly defined the dilemma as being about 'the powers of a parent, the duties of a doctor and the rights of a child'. In order to give valid independent consent which does not need validation (or knowledge) by the parents, the (underage) child must be 'of sufficient intellect and maturity to understand fully the nature of what is being proposed'. This does not, however, automatically deprive the parents/guardians of their right to determine treatment for their child (if under 18), and in cases of conflict it may be necessary to seek wardship jurisdiction[35,36], which has the ultimate legal redress. Further-more, it is left to the doctor to decide whether the child is competent or not.

This spirit of emerging autonomy through childhood was embodied in the subsequent Children Act of 1989. Complications however exist with dissent or refusal of treatment by the child which, although the logical opposite of consent and subject to the same criteria of capacity and under-standing as for an adult, can be legally overridden by parents or wardship jurisdiction (as in the case of Re W[36]). Information giving is of course the key to obtaining consent. This should always involve children, informing them at an appropriate level of understanding for their age while also lis-tening to, and taking into account, their views. Such an approach is encap-sulated by the statement from the Royal College of Paediatrics and Child Health (RCPCH) that 'good practice goes beyond observing minimum legal standards and takes account of higher ethical standards of respect for children's views as well as concerns as to their welfare'[2]. It is also embodied in the Children Act[37] and the UN Convention of the Rights of the Child[38].

Can children/minors refuse treatment?

For adults, refusal is the counterpart of consent in the expression of their autonomy. But when the wishes of the family and the consent of the child or adolescent do not coincide, does the young person have a similar right to refuse[39]? The weight of influence a child's views are given in the decision making process must increase where the issue is one of quality rather than quantity of life, where it is an experimental rather than proven interven-tion which is being offered, where a child has prior knowledge of an illness or its treatment and where he/she is used to being consulted in the family context. In this case, it also depends on the child's concepts of near and far, and consideration not only of the child's best interests now but also those of the adult he will become, and how many close 'others' will be affected by the decision[1]. In all cases the process of consent must occur over time, and it is one of facilitating decision making. This process includes expert coun-seling, perhaps with appropriate visual and written information, and with 'every effort ... to elucidate the wishes of the patient in matters in which there is a choice'. This may require fostering an environment in which non-agreement is allowed and 'an understanding of (why) the young patient may decline to store spermatozoa, talking these reasons through and recording them'[40]. Positive aspects of such an approach include evidence that children who participate in clinical decisions pertaining to their treatment have a better and faster rate of recovery and psychological re-adjustment[41].

Predicting the future: the adults and potential parents children become

Meanwhile, while freezing oocytes remains difficult, and there is no certainty that ovarian tissue cryopreservation is effective either for obtaining gametes or as an autograft, single women or parents of adolescents have enquired whether oocytes might be stimulated and fertilized *in vitro* as embryos using donor sperm. Specific ethical dilemmas pertain to the freezing of embryos, especially with respect to the duration of cryopreservation and their ultimate fate[42], while the use of donor sperm further complicates this issue[43]. Such decisions are usually, though by no means exclusively, made in the context of a long-term adult partnership and where male sterility is absolute and incurable. Here again varied European legislative approaches to the treatment of single women reflect different ethical appraisals of the reproductive rights of women and the welfare or interest of the unborn child. In the UK the Human Fertilisation and Embryology Authority (HFEA) Code of Practice[44] mentions the need to consider the father as a factor when judging the welfare of the future child. It is impossible to predict the future pragmatic and moral position of a young woman wishing to accomplish the reproductive plans made years earlier with the contribution of donated gametes.

The proposal described by Bahadur and colleagues in the context of sperm freezing[40] seems indeed appropriate: it entails the type of issues which should be discussed by clinicians before referral to the sperm storage laboratory, including the possible need for ART, the possible chances of success or failure and the concern that any such future therapy may not receive state funding. Although it is good practice to enroll the support of parents if the child so wishes, procreation is an instance of a reproductive right in English law[14], and only a 'competent' patient, even though underage, may sign the form for gamete storage, use and disposal. Thus children will need to address issues of gamete use (for research or procreation) and disposal in the event of their death or mental incapacitation and have their understanding of these issues tested.

By contrast, gonadal tissue may not necessarily contain gametes under the definition of the HFEA ('a reproductive cell ... which has a haploid set of chromosomes and which is able to take part in fertilisation with another of the opposite sex to form a zygote'[45]), and thus, despite its reproductive intent, through a potential legal loophole, can be removed by proxy consent under common law[46,47]. If the child eventually dies of his or her initial or relapsed disease, before he/she reaches an age of maturity sufficient to revisit the consent, establish a sexual relationship or consider reproduction, provision must be made to deal with the outcome of any frozen gonadal tissues. Might the parents have any access to the gametes that represent the only life potential of their dead child at a time of overwhelming grief?

After the lengthy debates and court involvement of the Blood case[48], another case is currently making headlines in the UK. A young man who had agreed to the posthumous use of his sperm by his girlfriend has died and she has made clear her lack of interest in the matter. His parents are trying to obtain access to the samples although this would be in total contradiction to the HFE Act consent provisions, which require prior written consent for posthumous use from the partner and not the relatives. One might argue that procreation outside the context of the couple, decided by potential grandparents rather than parents, is not compatible with the requirement for consideration of the welfare of the future child as stated by the HFE Act 1990 nor in the spirit of the Children Act 1989, which places emphasis on parental responsibility to their children rather than parental rights. The code of practice of the HFEA lists factors to be taken into account with regard to the welfare of the child. These include (the parents') commitment to having and bringing up a child or children and their ability to provide a stable and supportive environment for any child produced as a result of treatment, their medical histories and the medical histories of their families as well as their age and future ability to look after or provide for a child's need amongst others. This latter requirement alone may well preclude grandparents commissioning, for instance, a surrogate mother to be inseminated with their deceased son's sperm. This poignant problem is one of many which confirms the need for a firmer protection of the interests of the children and adolescents concerned. It is suggested that parental responsibility is limited to safe keeping of tissues[49] (storage only) and precludes the use of created gametes for the purpose of procreation in the event of death or mental incapacitation.

Ethical issues: for whose benefit, if not the child's?

The complexity of the problem is illustrated by the consensus statement of a 3-day meeting in the UK in Dec 1999[50] convened 'to develop an ethically acceptable strategy for practice and research into preserving fertility of children and young people being treated for cancer'. The Late Effects Committee of the UK Children's Cancer Study Group (UKCCSG)[51] points out that the 'need for follow up (and long term) strategies', as well as giving accurate and unbiased information without undue pressure or coercion, is one of the elements of obtaining consent. The essence of the pediatrician's professional practice is underpinned by a requirement to act always 'in the child's best interests and have a duty of care beyond the minimum legal requirement'[2]. Indeed the intent, the conservation of the reproductive ability of children and adolescents, seems *prima facie* beneficent, but it may sometimes reflect the wish of the young sufferer's parents and not his/her own, while it certainly has implications for many other autonomous people, in particular their future partner. The parental decision may be biased by an unconscious desire to one day have a grandchild, which might predominate over their child's views/best interest at the time. This may further be complicated by the fact that ovarian biopsy may indeed be a fairly risky procedure in a relatively sick adolescent female, much more so than sperm donation and, unlike the latter, with no proven chance of success.

While the treatment of males or the repair, in the psychoanalytical sense, of the couple's infertility by artificial insemination of frozen thawed sperm is current practice, it may be argued that cryopreservation of prepubertal testicular and ovarian tissues is still in the research phase, as indeed are the techniques of gametes maturation *in vitro*, or tissues autograft. The consent one needs to obtain from the patient is thus of a different kind, being further complicated by the distinction between therapeutic and non-therapeutic research. The definition of therapeutic research is one which carries benefit for the patient, usually understood as a more or less immediate benefit for a current condition. It is common practice in the area of pediatric oncology, where therapeutic advances and increases in survival rates could not otherwise have been achieved. Virtually any procedure might be justified on these terms but it is not usually applicable to events in the distant future in which further untested therapeutic intervention will be required, as in our dilemma. This highlights the problems of obtaining consent from children for future situations[52] and the reasons why this should be a staged process as already advocated for the use of human tissue for research purposes[53]. Long-term follow-up of outcome is also essential, especially in order to decide if and when the line between research and therapy has been crossed and a technique may be offered more routinely to young patients.

Finally we must not forget that there is always the problem of distributive justice in a context where resources are limited. Several studies show the lack of priority the public attribute to infertility, which affects some 12% of healthy couples. What then should we make of the even less immediate problem of fertility preservation of children whose lifespan may be reduced, whose potential life-saving therapy may be delayed by experimental attempts to preserve a function which is not life-limiting, may not be definitely impaired and in which alternative future treatment strategies may exist for consideration when adult, and after stable partnerships are formed (ICSI, OD). It is possible that society would actually decide to provide the finances for storage for these vulnerable children, but be reluctant to shoulder the financial burden of actual treatment later on when feasible, in a doubly iniquitous approach already well described[54].

CONCLUSION

The UKCCSG urges a voluntary code of practice 'in order to ensure safety in this area, with specific consideration of: (1) which group of minors should be offered opportunities for fertility protection, and which group should not; (2) which harvest and storage methods are most appropriate; (3) how valid consent is best obtained; and (4) the possible role of the HFEA in regulating this activity'. Because of the sensitivity needed for these decisions, counseling should play a major role in the process of obtaining consent. Because of the responsibility we collectively hold towards children, wider discussion and consultation need to take place, and this is currently ongoing in the UK under the auspices of the British Fertility Society working group. The HFE Act includes the provision of counseling in reproductive decisions and protects the interests of patients by ensuring that adequate information is offered and proper consent obtained, and it would therefore seem appropriate in the UK that vulnerable young cancer sufferers should be offered the same rights and protection over their future reproductive potential.

That for the time being the definition of the word 'gametes' means that only postpubertal males are protected by legislation, exemplifies the semantic difficulties of legal interpretation of biological definitions. We need to protect the most vulnerable members of society, who undergo an invasive procedure for gonadal tissue collection under the common law of consent despite its intended reproductive use. As the HFE Act 1990 is considered a good model, able to protect the patient in most instances, thought should be given to the possible revision of the terminology in the legislation in order to include the same regulations for immature gametes as well as for mature gametes. The term reproductive tissues, or a redefinition of gametes to include both mature and immature cells, might help to close the present legal loophole in order to protect both our young patients and their offspring. It seems appropriate to hope that the same storage regulations for immature as well as for mature gametes will be applied in the UK. This would protect both patient and offspring and ensure that society as a whole is concerned with the well-being of young patients with cancer.

REFERENCES

1. Lansdown R. Listening to children: have we gone too far (or not far enough?). *J R Soc Med* 1998;91:457–8
2. The Royal College of Paediatrics and Child Health. *Withholding or Withdrawing Life-Saving Treatment in Children. A Framework for Practice*. London, Royal College of Paediatrics and Child Health, 1997
3. Hawkins MM, Smith RA. Pregnancy outcomes in childhood cancer survivors: probable effects of abdominal irradiation. *Int J Cancer* 1989;43:399–402
4. Meadows AT, Hobbie WL. The medical consequences of cure. *Cancer* 1986; 58:524–8
5. Grundy R, Gosden RG, Hewitt M, *et al*. Fertility preservation for children treated for cancer (1): scientific advances and research dilemmas. *Arch Dis Child* 2001;84:355–9
6. Sanders JE, Hawley J, Levy W, *et al*. Pregnancies following high dose cyclophosphamide with or without high-dose busulphan or total body irradiation and bone marrow transplantation. *Blood* 1996;87:3045–52
7. Apperley JF, Reddy N. Mechanisms and management of treatment-related gonadal failure in recipients of high-dose chemotherapy. *Blood Rev* 1995;9: 93–116
8. Ash P. The influence of radiation on fertility in man. *Br J Radiol* 1980;53: 271–8
9. Critchley HOD, Wallace WHB, Shalet SM, *et al*. Abdominal irradiation in childhood; the potential for pregnancy. *Br J Obstet Gynaecol* 1992;99:392–4
10. Bath LE, Critchley HOD, Chambers SE, *et al*. Ovarian and uterine characteristics after total body irradiation in childhood and adolescence. *Br J Obstet Gynaecol* 1999;106:1265–72
11. Otkay R, Karlikaya G. Ovarian function after transplantation of frozen, banked autologous ovarian tissue. *N Engl J Med* 2000;342:1919
12. Radford JA, Lieberman BA, Brison DR, *et al*. Orthotopic reimplantation of cryopreserved ovarian cortical strips after high-dose chemotherapy for Hodgkin's lymphoma. *Lancet* 2001;357:1172–5
13. Schover LR. Psychosocial aspects of infertility and decisions about reproduction in young cancer survivors: a review. *Med Pediatr Oncol* 1999;33:53–9
14. *The Human Fertilisation and Embryology Act 1990*. London: HMSO, 1990
15. Chapman RM, Sutcliffe SB, Rees LH, *et al*. Cyclical combination chemotherapy and gonadal function. Retrospective study in males. *Lancet* 1979;1:285–9
16. Vigersky RA, Chapman RM, Berenberg J, Glass AR. Testicular dysfunction in untreated Hodgkin's disease. *Am J Med* 1982;73:482–6
17. Jorgensen M, Keiding N, Skakkebaek NE. Estimation of spermarche from longitudinal spermaturia data. *Biometrics* 1991;47:177–93
18. Nielsen CT, Skakkebaek NE, Richardson DW, *et al*. Onset of the release of spermatozoa (spermarche) in boys in relation to age, testicular growth, pubic hair, and height. *J Clin Endocrinol Metab* 1986;62:532–5
19. Spoudeas HA, Wallace WHB, Walker D. Is germ cell harvest and storage justified in minors treated for cancer? *Br Med J* 2000;320:316

20. Meistrich ML, Wilson G, Brown BW, *et al*. Impact of cyclophosphamide on the long-term reduction in sperm count in men treated with combination therapy for Ewing and soft tissue sarcomas. *Cancer* 1992;70:2703–12

21. Tournaye H, Liu j, Nagy Z, *et al*. Correlation between testicular histology and outcome after ICSI using testicular sperm. *Hum Reprod* 1996;11:127–32

22. Baker TG. Radiosensitivity of mammalian oocytes with particular reference to the human female. *Am J Obstet Gynecol* 1971;110(5):746–61

23. Wallace W, Shalet SM, Hendry JH, *et al*. Ovarian failure following abdominal irradiation in childhood: the radiosensitivity of the human oocyte. *Br J Radiol* 1989;62:995–8

24. Chapron C, Querleu D, Bruhat MA, *et al*. Surgical complications of diagnostic and operative gynaecological laparoscopy: a series of 29,966 cases. *Hum Reprod* 1998;13:867–72

25. Otkay K, Newton H, Aubard Y, *et al*. Cryopreservation of immature human oocytes and ovarian tissue: an emerging technology? *Fertil Steril* 1998;69:1–7

26. Fabbri R, Porcu E, Marsella T, *et al*. Human oocyte cryopreservation: new perspectives regarding oocyte survival. *Hum Reprod* 2001;16:411–16

27. Chian RC, Buckett WM, Too LL, Tan SL. Pregnancies resulting from in vitro matured oocytes retrieved from patients with polycystic ovary syndrome after priming with human chorionic gonadotropin. *Fertil Steril* 1999; 72(4):639–42

28. Shaw JM, Bowles J, Koopman P, *et al*. Fresh and cryopreserved ovarian tissue samples from donors with lymphoma transmit the cancer to graft recipients. *Hum Reprod* 1996;11:1668–73

29. Kim SS, Radford J, Harris M, *et al*. Ovarian tissue harvested from lymphoma patients to preserve fertility may be safe for autotransplantation. *Hum Reprod* 2001;16:2056–60

30. HFEA 10th annual report 1999, HFEA, London, 2000

31. Weil E. Le secret pour qui? *Contracept Fertil Sex* 1992;20(7–8):737–40

32. Declaration of the World Medical Association Helsinski (1964, as amended in 1975 and 1983)

33. The Family Law Reform Act 1969. London: HMSO, 1969

34. *Gillick vs West Norfolk and Wisbech Area Health Authority* (1986). Appeal cases 112–207

35. *Re R* (1991) 4 All ER 177

36. *Re W* (1992) 4 All ER 627

37. *Children's Act, 1989*. London: HMSO, 1989

38. UN Convention on the Rights of the Child /www.freethechildren.org/UNCRC.htm

39. Devereux JA, Jones DPH, Dickenson DI. Can children withhold consent to treatment? *Br Med J* 1993;306:1459–61

40. Bahadur G, Whelan J, Ralph D, Hindmarsh P. Gaining consent to freeze spermatozoa from adolescents with cancer: legal, ethical and practical aspects. *Hum Reprod* 2001;16:188–93

41. Cooklin AI. Tenderness and toughness in the face of distress. *Palliat Med* 1989; 3:89–95

42. Cryopreservation of embryos, ESHRE Taskforce on ethics and law. *Hum Reprod* 2001;16:1049–50

43.   Shenfield F, Steele SJ. What are the effects of anonymity and secrecy on the welfare of the child in gamete donation? *Hum Reprod* 1997;12:392–5

44.   *HFEA Code of Practice*, 5th edn. London: HFEA, 2001

45.   Storage of testicular tissue, CMO's update 17, Department of Health, Feb 1998

46.   Hewitt M, Walker DA, Sokal M. Human Fertilisation and Embryology Act 1990 discriminates against children. *Br Med J* 1998;317:543

47.   Deech R. Human Fertilisation and Embryology Act 1990 discriminates against children. *Br Med J* 1998;316:1095

48.   *R v. Human Fertilisation and Embryology Authority ex parte Diane Blood* (1997)

49.   Bahadur G, Chatterjee R, Ralph D. Testicular tissue cryopreservation in boys. Ethical and legal issues. *Hum Reprod* 2000;15(6):1416–20

50.   Wallace WHB, Walker DA. Conference consensus statement: ethical and research dilemmas for fertility preservation in children treated for cancer. *Hum Fertil* 2001;4:69–76

51.   Wallace WHB, Blacklay A, Eiser C, *et al.*, on behalf of the late effects committee of the United Kingdom Children's Cancer Study Group. Developing strategies for long term follow up of survivors of childhood cancer. *Br Med J* 2001;323:271–4

52.   Dickenson D. Can children and young people consent to be tested for adult genetic disorders? *Br Med J* 1998;318:1063–6

53.   *Human Tissue. Ethical and Legal Issues*. London: Nuffield Council on Bioethics, 1995

54.   Shenfield F. Justice and access to fertility treatments. In: Shenfield F and Sureau C, eds. *Ethical Dilemmas in Assisted Reproduction*. Carnforth, UK: Parthenon Publishing, 1997:7–14

3

Providing infertility treatment to HIV-positive people: considerations regarding the moral responsibility of the physician

G. Pennings

INTRODUCTION

It will take time before the general attitude towards procreation by HIV-positive people changes. Since it became known that the virus was transmitted from mother to child, infected mothers were urged to abstain from procreation. Several factors combined to bring about this attitude: the severity of the disease, fear and uncertainty about the spread of the epidemic, negative status of the most affected groups (intravenous drug users and homosexuals) etc. In the meantime, many things have changed. However, the initial cognitive scheme of the disease, on which the negative attitude was based, tends to ignore dissonant information. Nevertheless, the accumulation of new developments forces people to reconsider the scheme of AIDS and indirectly the moral rules and recommendations based on it[1-3]. Two major elements, mainly due to improved treatment methods, are important for the present discussion: the considerable increase in the life expectancy of HIV-infected persons and the significant reduction of the perinatal transmission of the virus. As a consequence, more and more HIV-infected people start thinking about building a family.

This chapter concentrates on the question whether fertility specialists should help HIV-infected people to have children. Although this question is related to the question whether HIV-infected persons should forgo childbearing (as we will discuss), the distinction should be kept in mind. The essential difference is the contribution by the physician. When people can have children without any external help, they are personally responsible for the outcome. When the intervention of others is needed, the standards change. Parents are allowed to take certain reproductive risks but this does not imply that others should go along. If we transferred our question to genetic diseases, the question would be whether people (fertile or infertile) with a high risk of transmitting a genetic disease should get access to assisted reproductive technology.

BRINGING CHILDREN INTO THE WORLD AND EVALUATING THEIR INTERESTS

Responsible parenthood refers to the considerations and circumstances that couples should take into account when contemplating whether or not to conceive. Most people agree that the well-being of their future child should be the primary concern of prospective parents[4]. However, what this means in practice differs considerably for each individual. A fundamental contradiction in the general attitude toward parental control in reproduction is demonstrated on risk-taking. On the one hand, one condemns parents who have all possible preimplantation or prenatal tests in order to guarantee that the child will be healthy. On the other hand, parents who take certain risks are blamed for being selfish and for putting their own desires and wishes above the interests of the child. The intermediate position would be that couples should avoid having children if there is a foreseeable high risk that the future child will have a serious disease or handicap[5].

In ethics, avoiding actions which cause harm to others is one of the most fundamental principles. To determine the acceptability of a decision or action, two crucial elements are considered: the magnitude and the probability of the harm. Feinberg[6] observed that the variation between magnitude and probability of harm can be expressed in a concise formula: 'the greater the gravity of the envisioned harm, the less probable it need be'. The harm principle applied to the question of reproductive responsibility says that 'the greater the magnitude and probability of predicted harm, the less justifiable it is to have children'[7].

Gravity of the illness

AIDS and the welfare of the child

Everybody agrees on the fundamental importance of the welfare of the children when judging the acceptability of new reproductive technologies. Most medical associations have issued statements in this regard. However, the practical utility of the rule is fairly limited. The first problem is the general difficulty of calculating the quality of life of a person. This problem is aggravated by the special difficulty in procreation, i.e. the need to predict the quality of life of future persons. The second problem concerns the evaluation of the quality of life. Even if we manage to calculate and quantify the quality of life, we would still need to agree on a standard to judge what amount is acceptable. Three evaluation rules can be found in the literature:

(1) the maximal welfare, (2) the reasonable welfare and (3) the minimal threshold[8].

The maximal welfare rule states that parents should not knowingly and intentionally bring a child into the world in less than ideal circumstances. This is an extremely strong standard and the consistent application of this rule would exclude the overwhelming majority of the population from procreation. Nevertheless this standard has been used to refuse access to infertility treatment to lesbian couples and older postmenopausal women[9]. According to some, children should ideally be raised by a mother and a father. Families which deviate from the heterosexual nuclear family are considered a less than optimal environment for the upbringing of children. A similar argument is advanced regarding the ideal parent. Certain characteristics of would-be parents (like being poor, obese, workaholic etc.) are seen as detrimental and harmful to the psychological and social development of the child. Consequently, people with these characteristics should refrain from procreation and *a fortiori* should not be assisted in the realization of their wish to have a child. However, there are no reliable predictive criteria for adequate parenting, and consequently no criteria to guarantee the best interests of the child[10].

At the other end of the spectrum lies the minimal threshold. The overwhelming majority of the authors discussing the problem of the acceptability of bringing persons into the world adopts this standard. The standard is also known as the 'wrongful life' or 'worse than death' standard: 'a child should not be brought into the world if and only if its life quality is so low that it would have been better never to have been born at all'[11,12]. This is an extremely low standard which again leads to strong counter-intuitive judgments. On this account, it is not even possible to say that it is wrong to bring a child into existence whose prospects and opportunities are awful[13]. Applied to procreative decisions by HIV-positive persons, it would not be wrong to conceive knowingly and intentionally an HIV-positive child. Not all infected children are seriously ill and expected to survive only a few years at best[14]. Two categories of children can be distinguished: those who develop AIDS within the first two years of life and those who survive into older childhood or early adolescence. The majority of the children will remain asymptomatic during their elementary school years. With the new antiretroviral therapy, the time from infection to the development of AIDS will lengthen substantially. So although these children have a strongly reduced life expectancy, the life they have is not characterized by unbearable suffering from the beginning until the end. The typical scenario 'involves years of recurrent and progressively more complex health problems, finally ending with death'[14]. Only about the children who develop AIDS within the first year and die soon after could it be argued that their life is not worth living and that they would have been better off not being born at all[7].

Finally, the third standard to evaluate the application of the new reproductive technologies has been introduced as a way to avoid the counter-intuitive judgments of the two other rules[8]. According to this standard the provision of medical assistance is acceptable when the child born as a result of the treatment will have a reasonably happy life. Although different definitions can be found as to what constitutes a decent welfare level, the common core of most definitions is that a person has a decent quality of life when he or she has the abilities and opportunities to realize those dimensions and aspects that in general make human life valuable. An important obstacle for children born HIV-infected to have a decent quality of life is the strongly reduced life expectancy. When a child can hope to live to its twenties at most, there is very little time left for a family or a career. This makes the realization of the majority of important life plans simply impossible. Add to this the effects of the illness (repeated hospitalization, side-effects of the medication) and the probable experience of parental death (possibly combined with other major life changes) and one ends up with an expected quality of life that is below the reasonable level.

Reduced parental life expectancy

Parental death is an element which is largely ignored in the discussion. One tends to concentrate on medical risks while ignoring the broader social and psychological context in which the risks and the consequences are interpreted and lived by the people involved. There is a general agreement that the death of a parent is one of the most devastating traumas a child can experience[15]. The disruption of the social structure connected to the loss of the parent as a primary caretaker may have profound effects on the child's later social and emotional development. But the parental life expectancy also raises more philosophical questions about the meaning of parenthood. Is it reasonable to want to have children when one knows that one will not be able to raise them and to see them grow up? Is the right to procreate worth defending and supporting when it only covers the right to beget and bear a child without child rearing and upbringing? These questions were also raised when the acceptability of postmenopausal motherhood was debated. Parenthood is conceived as a long-term commitment. Parents commit themselves to a whole range of obligations by virtue of their decision to bear offspring. Although there may be legitimate reasons to separate the genetic, gestational and rearing aspects of parenting, the decision to bring a child into the world brings with it a *prima facie* duty to take care of the child[16]. This implies that parents should expect to live until the child is approximately 18[17]. Until now HIV-infected people could not have expected to live long enough to discharge their parental obligations. However, as for postmenopausal women, this argument shows another largely implicit principle, namely that intending parents should be able to raise their child alone. Women with AIDS will become more seriously ill and they will experience prolonged periods of incapacity. The parents' ability to care for the child will be seriously compromised long before their death. They should not only live until the child reaches adulthood but also remain competent to provide care and guidance for approximately 18 years. The long-term aspect of the commitment is sometimes ignored because the reliance on medical technology needed to achieve the pregnancy focuses attention on the condition of the parents at the time of conception and birth.

The parent's ability to provide the daily care of the child can be sustained by supportive services[18]. In essence, the question is to what extent society is prepared to support parents who show a reduced capacity because of illness or handicap. Indirectly, this willingness expresses the value attached to the right to procreate and the sincere concern for the welfare of children born in less then optimal circumstances. It could be argued that the parents do not necessarily have to be available for the child if only they planned arrangements for substitute parenting in case one or both die or become incapacitated[19]. Nevertheless, if a parental project is started by a couple, at least one of them should expect to be able to raise the child. For this reason, the intention of couples to create offspring should not be supported if both partners are HIV positive. Transferring the parental commitment to other family members or good friends should only be considered as a solution when the child is already born. In other words it is a back-up measure in case things go wrong, not a sufficient reason to justify planning a pregnancy. In a similar vein, some assert that the advances in HIV treatment do not remove the objections to provide infertility treatment. They claim that the medical measures to prevent perinatal transmission should be seen as 'useful advice on how to minimize the likelihood of a tragic outcome given a dangerous or high-risk situation that already exists. It would be a flawed leap in judgment to extend automatically the study results to justify creating dangerous situations'[20].

Probability of the illness

The second factor needed to estimate the risk beside the magnitude and gravity of the illness is the probability that harm will occur. Here a distinction should be made according to the sex of the seropositive partner. When the male partner is seropositive, the chance of infecting his partner and indirectly his offspring is very low if all precautions are respected. Although the evidence is not conclusive at this moment, the data provided by clinics in Italy and Spain who used washed sperm for artificial insemination are promising. After a few thousand cycles of insemination and a few hundred births, not one seroconversion has been observed[21,22]. These data llow the conclusion to be reached that medical assistance can help these men to have genetically-related uninfected children.

The most important consideration, however, is the mother–child transmission rate. While at the beginning of the epidemic vertical transmission was around 20% in European countries, the introduction of zidovudine in 1994 brought the risk down to 8%. New antiretroviral therapies and a number of other measures like scheduled caesarean deliveries have further reduced the overall transmission rate to below 2%[3,23]. The acceptability of risk is something about which reasonable people will disagree. There is no moral theory sufficiently precise and elaborate to determine exact numbers of acceptable risk[7,24].

COMPLICITY IN THE REALIZATION OF THE PARENTAL PROJECT

We start from the premise that the fertility specialist is an accessory or collaborator of the parents, who should be considered as the principals. The physician has to decide whether he will participate in the parental project of the intending parents. This structure explains in part the particular situation in which he finds himself. On the one hand, he makes a judgment on what the parents can or should do and the risks they are allowed to take. On the other hand, he contributes to the outcome of the treatment as a causal agent and thus is accountable for the result. This implies that the doctor must make a normative judgment about the rightness of his act[25]. This generates the possibility of a discrepancy between the evaluation of the parents' decision and the evaluation of his own contribution. Since his decision to participate is voluntary and deliberate, he engages himself as a moral agent and thus blocks the possibility of 'hiding' completely behind the requesting parents. In other words, he cannot reduce himself to a mere instrument. He does not have to share the values of the parents but he should be able to justify his own participation.

Which judgment should he follow? In ethics we distinguish between different categories of actions. Actions can be morally required or obligatory, morally recommendable, bad but morally permissible and morally forbidden[24]. Since most people consider moral principles as absolute and universal, the category 'bad but morally permissible' frequently leads to misunderstandings. It is partially based on the acceptance of moral pluralism in society. We should accept that some actions which we consider wrong from our moral point of view should nevertheless be permitted because people with alternative moral codes may judge these actions differently. Engelhardt expressed this as follows: 'X has a moral right to do A, but it is wrong'[26]. The main problem for the physician is to draw a line between 'bad but permissible' and impermissible. Other dimensions that interfere with the modalities of moral action are the acts/omissions and the positive rights/negative rights. Permissible is generally interpreted as 'n action should be taken to prevent the exercise of the right'. The negative right to procreate of HIV-positive persons would be violated by forced contraception or sterilization. However, infertile persons do not have a positive right to medical assistance. Nevertheless, we think that infertile people in normal circumstances should be helped to realize what is considered an important life plan. Two powerful arguments are presented to respect the wishes of the parents by helping them: the duty of care of the medical profession and the autonomy of a person to lead his or her life according to his or her own value system and moral code. These arguments shift the burden of proof: a physician should justify why he will not help a couple to procreate. Given the doctors' monopoly position in offering help[27], a refusal to help an infertile couple in reality comes down to a denial of their right to procreate. The doctor has control responsibility because of his technical skills and medical knowledge[28]. The childlessness of the rejected woman is thus also a consequence of a decision by the physician and not simply the course of nature. Not helping a sterile couple is equally effective in obstructing the realization of the wish as sterilizing a fertile couple. Although the violation of a negative right is generally considered more serious than the violation of a positive right, it could be argued that the morally relevant point is not whether it happens by an act or omission but whether there is a willful obstruction of a right. In my opinion, physicians should only refuse collaboration if the wish is evaluated as 'impermissible'. This would be the case if rational persons would accept that the risk of having a child who will not have a reasonably happy life is too high. A tolerant attitude and openness toward other values and principles when deciding this issue is highly recommended.

RISK-TAKING AND RECKLESSNESS

A physician who helps a couple to become pregnant is responsible for the welfare of the children that will be born. Of course, his responsibility is limited to foreseen (or foreseeable) consequences. When a child is born with a handicap, the fertility specialist is co-responsible as a collaborator. However, responsibility does not mean blameworthiness or culpability[29]. To determine his culpability, we have to analyze his actions. Let us look at natural reproduction for a start. The base rate of major malformations in the population is between 3 and 5%. Of every 100 children born, between three and five will have a serious handicap. This is equally true for all children born by means of medically assisted procreation. The morally important point is whether the assisting physician ought to be blamed for the results. It is obvious that no direct intention is involved. No physician in his right mind intends to create an HIV-infected child or a child with a handicap. The absence of direct intention, however, does not imply that no moral guilt is involved. People can be blamed not only for what they intend to bring about but also for what they intentionally bring about, i.e. for the consequences of which the person is morally certain that they will occur. For instance, if the doctor decides to administer a drug to a group of 100 patients when he knows the drug will cure 95 but will probably kill or make seriously ill the other five, he is responsible for the illness or death of the latter five persons. These five deaths are an unintended and unavoidable side-effect but they still are consequences of his intentional action. The moral importance of the difference is that those consequences are not part of one's chain of reasons for acting[30]. The doctor knows that these consequences will follow but he does not act in order to bring them about. Instead of arguing that foresight entails intentionality, and intentionality entails responsibility, we skip the intermediate step and argue that foresight is a sufficient condition for responsibility[31]. Since a doctor knows the base rate in advance, he creates the risk of that harm intentionally. He at least accepted the possibility of the actualization of the harm. We condemn risk-taking as reckless when the person is aware of the risk but still goes ahead. 'Recklessness is conscious and unjustified risk-taking'[32]. Whether a risk is reasonable or not depends on the balance of its disvalue (magnitude of harm × probability) with the positive value it creates. It seems that a risk of serious harm in less than 5% of births is not considered unreasonable.

The most general justification for causing harm to other people is by pointing to the good that is generated by the same act: helping 95 healthy children to be born outweighs the cost and harm to the five children who are born with a handicap. The fact that there is no reasonable way at present to reduce this number plays an important role in this argument. The principle of proportionality states that the good which is sought must more than compensate for the bad effect. So the fact that the bad was not intended would not be sufficient to justify causing harm even for those who defend the doctrine of the double effect[33]. The good also needs to outweigh the bad. Two other conditions can be added: that there should exist no alternative which brings about a better balance and that there be no acceptable way to diminish the harm.

The dilemma is brought about by the wish to help infertile people to have children. This cannot be done without also bringing into the world children with a handicap. The 'safest' solution would be not to help people to have children. This would annihilate the risk completely but of course no children would be born to infertile couples. Auroux[34] argues concerning HIV-positive infertile couples that 'it seems shocking and unreasonable to me that medicine would intervene to restore a risk that was eliminated by nature' (my translation). However, this argument applies to all medical assistance offered to infertile couples. If it is acceptable to help HIV-negative couples to have children knowing that 3 to 5% of the children will have a major malformation, is it then completely unacceptable to help HIV-positive couples to have children knowing that, in addition to the base rate, 2% of the children will be born infected? It could be argued that the comparison with the base rate of malformations is ill-conceived since this rate comprises a mix of thousands of relatively rare disorders. However, we do not systematically screen specific groups known to have a high risk and neither do we refuse them access to infertility treatment. The probability of a woman above the age of 38 having a child with chromosomal abnormalities exceeds the probability of perinatal infection in HIV-positive women[3]. If the same reasoning were applied as for HIV, we should deny access to fertility treatment to these women or we should accept them on the condition that they agree to have a prenatal test and to terminate the pregnancy if the fetus is affected. It is highly unlikely that society would impose this condition. Moreover, if we find the current risk for HIV unacceptable, we should screen all fertility patients in the population for the most common genetic disorders, like cystic fibrosis[35].

It is understandable that many physicians feel reluctant to participate in a process that might lead to the creation of an HIV-infected child. An intermediate solution would be to postpone infertility treatment for HIV-positive persons 'until there is a negligible risk of perinatal transmission and a significantly better prognosis for HIV-infected mothers'[36]. Still, one wonders whether doctors do not accept less risk-taking from their patients than from themselves. One may doubt the consistency of a physician who refuses to help HIV-positive women because they consider the risk to be unacceptably high and who simultaneously routinely replaces three (or more) embryos in each IVF cycle. Multiple pregnancies are the cause of a strong increase in obstetric complications, perinatal morbidity, congenital malformations, maternal and fetal mortality and long-term social, psychological and economic difficulties[37,38]. Moreover, multiple pregnancies are to a large extent iatrogenic problems generated by the wish to increase the pregnancy rate whereas the serostatus of the couple is a given. When the perinatal mortality rate of IVF twins (4.7%) and IVF triplets (8.2%)[39] is compared with the risk of HIV infection when all efforts are made to reduce vertical transmission (2%), it becomes difficult for fertility specialists to argue that the latter risk is unacceptable. The inconsistent application of the best interests of the child standard is a ubiquitous feature in the discussions of new applications in assisted reproduction. Owing to its vagueness, the standard is often abused to condemn those applications one does not like for other, less widely held moral reasons[40].

CAUSAL CONTRIBUTION

Physicians can perform a large range of acts when a couple present themselves for infertility treatment. A first option would be to offer non-invasive investigations to exclude the most obvious causes of infertility and to give the couple a realistic prognosis[41]. This step is useful to prevent unnecessary risky behavior on the part of the partners. Some HIV-positive women are reluctant to take antiretroviral medication because of possible teratogenic effects on the fetus should they become pregnant, although they cannot get pregnant owing to factors unknown to them. Other couples have unprotected sex while the sperm quality of the man is inadequate to obtain spontaneous conception. Another possibility is to provide information and to assist at other preliminary steps, like determining the fertile window or teaching couples how to practice self-insemination. All the restrictions on treatment are instigated by the wish to limit one's own contribution, and they express the moral uneasiness physicians experience when confronted with such requests. The physician sees it as a way to distance himself from the active management of the treatment[42].

This 'solution' raises the question as to which element (causation or intention) is necessary for culpability and blameworthiness. If causal contribution suffices, a physician who does not want to aid an HIV-infected couple to have a child is not allowed to perform all risk reducing actions since risk reduction is mostly obtained by increasing the chance of becoming pregnant. What kind of acts may a physician perform without being considered as an accomplice? Smith and colleagues thought that teaching the patients to inseminate rather than inseminating the patients themselves removes them from the outcome. At first sight, this at least restricts their personal contribution. They did not make the woman pregnant, they just provided the information (and possibly the instruments) which enabled her to get pregnant. However, providing information is also an act. It is something the doctor does and which contributes to the possible pregnancy. The main difference from full-blown treatment is that the final step which leads to the conception is made by the couple. But is this morally relevant? There is no consensus on this point. On the one hand, it could be argued that providing the means (broadly speaking information as well as drugs, instruments, etc.) does not necessarily constitute complicity. A gynecologist who performs a prenatal diagnosis and informs the couple of the presence of a genetic condition in the fetus enables the parents to decide to terminate the pregnancy. Thorp and colleagues[43] have argued that abortion is not the responsibility of the gynecologist who does the prenatal test. It is the patient who finally decides to abort or not. However, in the debate on sex selection, some people want to forbid telling the sex of the embryo or fetus to the parents in order to avoid a selection for sexist reasons. If providing information on a handicap does not turn the physician into an accessory to the termination of pregnancy, then why would this be the case when the doctor informs the parents about the sex of the fetus? It seems that a consistent attitude would pose a serious problem for gynecologists who do not want to be associated with terminations of pregnancy even when therapeutic abortions are considered.

INTENTION OR FORESIGHT?

In the philosophical literature a discussion is going on about whether the intention of the physician plays a role in the moral evaluation of his collaboration. According to one side, the physician can only be considered an accomplice, and consequently will only be blameworthy, if he acts with the intention to help the parents to realize their wish. In normal circumstances this is evidently the case: the doctor intends to help the couple to procreate. However, the same acts of medical assistance can also be performed without this intention. The doctor can help the couple to get pregnant without having the intention of helping them to become pregnant. The Gillick case can clarify this reasoning. The Gillick case concerns the right of a physician to prescribe contraceptives to an underage girl. Having intercourse with a girl under sixteen is a criminal offence in the United Kingdom. If the physician prescribes contraceptives, does he become an accomplice to unlawful sexual intercourse? Different opinions are brought forward: for some, the doctor is liable because he knows that the offence is likely to be committed and because he knows that the provision of contraceptives is likely to assist or encourage its commission. Knowledge of these issues combined with a voluntary act of participation is sufficient to prove the intention to aid and abet[44]. However, the majority of the Lords disagreed. They argued that the doctor would not be guilty if he did not intend to aid the girl to have sex but only acted to protect her against the possible harmful effects (pregnancy, sexually transmitted diseases) of intercourse.

Which alternative reasons could the physician supply to justify his collaboration beside the wish to help the parents to procreate? One acceptable alternative is the wish to protect the best interests of the couple and indirectly of the child. This reason relies on the fact that some fertile couples demand medical assistance in order to reduce the risk of infection for partner and offspring. In the case of fertile couples, the doctor providing medical assistance to a fertile HIV-positive couple to have a child does not have to intend to help them to have a child. This assertion conflicts with Chisholm's position that 'if a rational man acts with the intention of bringing about a certain state of affairs p and if he believes that by bringing about p he will bring about the conjunctive state of affairs, p and q, then he does act with the intention of bringing about p and q'[45]. A man who boards a plane to London does not need to have the intention of going to London. He knows with certainty that he will go to London but that does not mean that he intends to go there[46]. He might be boarding the first plane leaving Brussels because the Belgian police are looking for him. Of course, people normally infer that a person acted with the intention to bring about the consequences that are likely or highly probably to occur. If no alternative reasons are available, this is the most rational choice. However, foresight or knowledge of probable or even certain consequences is not the same as intention. So while the physician knows that teaching patients to self-inseminate or providing them with fertility drugs will help them to have a child, he can still claim that he does not intend to help them to become pregnant. His major reason for collaborating is risk reduction. The physician of course knows that, like the contraceptives for the under-age girl, his acceptance to assist may actually encourage and promote pro-creation by the couple. A number of HIV-discordant couples do not want to abandon safe sex to realize their wish to have a child for fear of infecting the HIV-negative partner[47]. Risk reduction is the necessary condition for these couples to start the project. However, contrary to the unlawful inter-course, having children by HIV couples is not wrong in itself. It is consid-ered wrong because of the risk of transmission of HIV.

The intention makes a difference for the deontological physician who thinks it is wrong or morally impermissible to help HIV-infected couples to have children. He can justify his assistance by mentioning his duty to pro-tect the health of the couple and the future child. Without the intention, he does not become an accomplice to a wrongful act and does not act against his conscience. However, he should only participate in assisting fertile couples or those who are thought to be fertile. The claim that he does not act in order to help the parents to procreate becomes untenable when the couple is infertile since the risk he intends to reduce is a consequence of hazardous behavior by the couple to get pregnant. If they are known to be infertile such behavior makes no sense.

NEGATIVE RESPONSIBILITY

The decision by a doctor not to assist an HIV-positive couple to have a child is not causally inert. A doctor is also responsible for the consequences of his decision not to accept a couple for treatment[28]. A person is negatively responsible for the occurrence of a state of affairs when that state of affairs obtains or something happens because an agent did not do something[29]. Williams defines this form of responsibility as 'the view that I am just as responsible for things I allow or fail to prevent as for things I bring about, even when one of the causal links is the intervening act of another agent'[48]. This view on responsibility may have far-reaching consequences for a phy-sician confronted with a request for help by fertile couples. Imagine the following situation: a couple with an HIV-positive woman comes to the doctor's office. They want his help to have a child. They tell him that if he refuses they will go ahead anyway and will try to conceive naturally. The doctor thinks that having children when the woman is HIV-positive is wrong. However, he also knows that by refusing the risk of horizontal transmission to the partner the risk of vertical transmission increases. The parents may decide to shun medical care for the rest of the pregnancy because they feel rejected or fear coercive intervention from the physician.

Suppose now, for the sake of the argument, that 100 couples present themselves at this clinic with the same request. The doctor knows that as a consequence of his refusal to treat, more men will get infected while trying for a child and many more children will become infected. Suppose that in the doctor's country the perinatal infection rate is 20% if the woman has no medical support and 2% when all precautions are taken. The doctor would become negatively responsible for 18 infected children who would not have been infected but for his refusal of treatment. If he accepts the assumption of positive responsibility for the creation of two children who will be born infected, he can save the lives of 18 other children.

Take Williams's famous example of 'Jim and the Indians'[48]: Jim arrives in a South American town where an army captain is about to kill a group of Indians to convince the others not to go on protesting. The captain makes him an offer as an honorary guest: if Jim agrees to kill one Indian himself, the captain will let off 19 other Indians. If Jim refuses to shoot an Indian, the captain will kill all 20. Kamm argued that in this kind of situation where the captain is responsible for making the positive result (fewer Indians killed) dependent on Jim's action, the captain has complete positive moral responsibility for the consequences of Jim's act[49]. Transferred to the 'doctor and the patients' case, the parents would have positive moral responsibility even for the two children who would be born infected with the help of the doctor. The negative consequences of the decision to procreate are charged to the parents because they made the offer. The parents ask the doctor for help in order to stop them from doing worse things. Of course, the physician can never know after accepting collaboration whether the couple would really have tried anyway. They might have changed their minds after his refusal. However, we cannot expect certainty: the doctor's collaboration is acceptable if the potential parents made it reasonably clear to him/her that they would go ahead. Nevertheless, the doctor cannot be held morally responsible for the final consequences (i.e. the children born infected) when his decision or choice is followed by an autonomous choice or decision by the couple. In other words, just as the captain does not have to kill the Indians if Jim refuses, the parents do not have to go ahead and conceive, with all the risks involved, if the doctor refuses. It cannot be said that the refusal by the physician provoked or caused the decision by the couple to go ahead. The causal chain between the doctor's decision and the birth of infected children is broken. The decision of the doctor is just part of the context in which the couples have to decide. After the refusal the question for them is, 'do we try to conceive even if the risk of infection is higher?' The doctor's refusal does not explain the couple's decision: rather they may decide to try in spite of the higher risk.

CONCLUSION

When no negligence on the part of the physician can be proven, the reproach that can be made is that he accepted the risk to help bring a child into the world that might be HIV infected. However, this choice is only reckless and the physician is only blameworthy if this risk-taking is unjustified and unreasonable. As argued above, this does not seem to be the case. If all measures are taken to reduce the risk of transmission, the risk falls within the range that is accepted in reproduction. However, this only means that HIV infection should no longer be considered as an *a priori* reason to refuse couples. It does not imply that all HIV-discordant couples should be accepted for infertility treatment regardless of the personal circumstances. Aggravating conditions like intravenous drug use may raise doubts on the parental capacities of the parent. The medical history of the patient may contain indications that the normal life expectancy will not apply to him or her. However, when we deliberate these points, we have already put aside the moral rule currently adopted by most fertility centers, namely that being HIV positive is an absolute exclusion criterion for medically assisted procreation.

REFERENCES

1. Anderson DJ. Assisted reproduction for couples infected with the human immunodeficiency virus type 1. *Fertil Steril* 1999;72:592–4
2. Englert Y, Van Vooren J-P, Place I, Liesnard C, Laruelle C, Delbaere A. ART in HIV-infected couples: has the time come for a change of attitude? *Hum Reprod* 2001;16:1309–15
3. Lyerly AD, Anderson J. Human immunodeficiency virus and assisted reproduction: reconsidering evidence, reframing ethics. *Fertil Steril* 2001;5:843–58
4. Callahan S. An ethical analysis of responsible parenthood. *Birth Defects* 1979;15:217–38
5. Jecker NS. Reproductive risk taking and the nonidentity problem. *Soc Theory Practice* 1987;13:219–35
6. Feinberg J. *The Moral Limits of the Criminal Law. Vol. 1. Harm to Others.* New York, Oxford: Oxford University Press, 1984
7. Arras JD. AIDS and reproductive decisions: having children in fear and trembling. *Milbank Q* 1990;68:353–82
8. Pennings G. Measuring the welfare of the child: in search of the appropriate evaluation principle. *Hum Reprod* 1999;14:1146–50
9. Editorial. Too old to have a baby? *Lancet* 1993;341:344–5
10. Harris J. Wrongful birth. In: Bromham DR, Dalton ME, Jackson JC, eds. *Philosophical Ethics in Reproductive Medicine*. Manchester, UK: Manchester University Press, 1990:156–70
11. Robertson JA. *Children of Choice: Freedom and the New Reproductive Technologies.* Princeton, NJ: Princeton University Press, 1994

12. Strong C, Schinfeld JS. The single woman and artificial insemination by donor. *J Reprod Med* 1984;29:293–9
13. Steinbock B, McClamrock R. When is birth unfair to the child? *Hastings Center Rep* 1994;24:15–21
14. Hutton N. Health prospects for children born to HIV-infected women. In: Faden RR, Kass NE, eds. *HIV, AIDS and Childbearing: Public Policy, Private Lives*. Oxford: Oxford University Press, 1996:63–77
15. Siegel K, Freund B. Parental loss and latency age children. In: Dane BO, Levine C, eds. *AIDS and the New Orphans: Coping with Death*. Westport, CT: Auburn House, 1994:43–58
16. O'Neill O. Begetting, bearing, and rearing. In: O'Neill O, Ruddick W, eds. *Having Children: Philosophical and Legal Reflections*. Oxford: Oxford University Press, 1979:25–38
17. Pennings G. Age and assisted reproduction. *Med Law* 1995;14:531–41
18. Anderson GR. Bereavement and the new guardians. In: Dane BO, Levine C, eds. *AIDS and the New Orphans: Coping with Death*. Westport, CT: Auburn House, 1994:121–32
19. Nolan K. Human immunodeficiency virus infection, women, and pregnancy. *Obstet Gynecol Clin N Am* 1990;17:651–68
20. Spike J, Greenlaw J. Case study: ethics consultation. *J Law Med Ethics* 1994; 2:347–50
21. Marina S, Marina F, Alcolea R, *et al*. Human immunodeficiency virus type 1-serodiscordant couples can bear healthy children after undergoing intrauterine insemination. *Fertil Steril* 1998;70:35–9
22. Semprini AE, Fiore S, Oneta M, *et al*. Assisted reproduction in HIV-discordant couples. *Hum Reprod* 1998;13 (abstract book) 1:89
23. Musoke PM, Mmiro FA. Prevention of HIV mother to child transmission: a review. *AIDS Rev* 2000;2:203–70
24. Buchanan A, Brock DW, Daniels N, Wikler D. *From Chance to Choice: Genetics & Justice*. Cambridge: Cambridge University Press, 2000
25. Savulescu J. Should doctors intentionally do less than the best? *J Med Ethics* 1999;25.121–6
26. Engelhardt HT Jr. *Bioethics and Secular Humanism: the Search for a Common Morality*. Philadelphia: Trinity Press International, 1991
27. Harris J. Doctors' orders, rationality and the good life: commentary on Savulescy. *J Med Ethics* 1999;25:127–9
28. Frey RG. Some aspects of the doctrine of double effect. *Can J Phil* 1975;5:259–83
29. Harris J. *The Value of Life*. London: Routledge, 1985
30. Moore M. Intentions and mens rea. In: Gavison R, ed. *Issues in Contemporary Legal Philosophy: the Influence of H.L.A. Hart*. Oxford: Clarendon Press, 1987:245–70
31. Miller AR. Foresight, intention and responsibility. *South J Phil* 1989;27:71–85
32. Duff RA. *Intention, Agency and Criminal Liability: Philosophy of Action and the Criminal Law*. Oxford: Blackwell, 1990
33. Chan DK. Intention and responsibility in double effect cases. *Ethic Theory Moral Pract* 2000;3:405–34

34.   Auroux M. Faut-il traiter l'infertilité chez les couples dont l'un des partenaires est séropositif? *Contracept Fertil Sex* 1999;27:118–20

35.   Lewis-Jones DI, Gazvani MR, Mountford R. Cystic fibrosis in infertility: screening before assisted reproduction. *Hum Reprod* 2000;15:2415–17

36.   Rizk B, Dill SR. Counselling HIV patients pursuing infertility investigation and treatment. *Hum Reprod* 1997;12:415–16

37.   Hazekamp J, Bergh C, Wennerholm U-B, Hovatta O, Karlstrom PO, Selbing A. Avoiding multiple pregnancies: considerations of new strategies. *Hum Reprod* 2000;15:1217–19

38.   Olivennes F. Double trouble: yes a twin pregnancy is an adverse outcome. *Hum Reprod* 2000;15:1663–5

39.   Lieberman B. An embryo too many? *Hum Reprod* 1998;13:2664–6

40.   Pennings G. Multiple pregnancies: a test case for the moral quality of medically assisted reproduction. *Hum Reprod* 2000;15:2466–9

41.   Olaitan A, Reid W, Mocroft A, McCarthy S, Johnson M. Infertility among human immunodeficiency virus-positive women: incidence and treatment dilemmas. *Hum Reprod* 1996;11:2793–6

42.   Smith JR, Forster GE, Kitchen VS, Hooi YS, Munday PE, Paintin DB. Infertility management in HIV positive couples: a dilemma. *Br Med J* 1991;302: 1447–50

43.   Thorp JM, Wells SR, Bowes WA, Cefalo RC. Integrity, abortion, and the pro-life perinatologist. *Hastings Center Rep* 1995;25:27–8

44.   Dennis IH. The mental element for accessories. In: Smith P, ed. *Criminal Law: Essays in Honour of J C Smith*. London: Butterworths, 1987:40–67

45.   Chisholm R. The structure of intention. *J Phil* 1970;67:633–47

46.   Simester AP. Moral certainty and the boundaries of intention. *Ox J Legal Stud* 1996;16:445–69

47.   Chrystie IL, Mullen JE, Braude PR, *et al*. Assisted conception in HIV discordant couples: evaluation of semen processing techniques in reducing HIV viral load. *J Reprod Immunol* 1998;41:301–6

48.   Williams B. A critique of utilitarianism. In: Smart JJC, Williams B, eds. *Utilitarianism: For and Against*. New York: Cambridge University Press, 1973

49.   Kamm FM. Responsibility and collaboration. *Phil Public Affairs* 1999;28: 169–204

4

Creating a child to save another: HLA matching of siblings by means of preimplantation genetic diagnosis

G. Pennings and I. Liebaers

INTRODUCTION

Every new technique has its proponents and its opponents. People's attitudes towards new developments are determined by a large number of very broad and vague background theories. The difference in attitude can be traced back to two competing views of technology. The 'optimistic' view believes in the ultimate benefit of scientific progress and trusts the discretion of society and the people involved to regulate the developments. The 'pessimistic' view is 'deeply concerned by the slippery slope leading from bona fide therapeutic applications of genetic engineering to eugenic practices'[1]. These two views can be recognized in the public reception of preimplantation genetic diagnosis (PGD). This technology has been developed to avoid the transmission of genetic diseases to the next generation. Its specificity lies in the fact that the diagnosis is performed on *in vitro* embryos before the implantation in the uterus of the woman. From the start PGD has been attacked as a dangerous step leading to aberrations. A well-tested method is used to discredit the technology: one states that PGD leads straight to eugenics. Instead of looking at the real applications, the opponents start making far-fetched speculations regarding possible future developments. However, it needs some explaining to link PGD for human leukocyte antigen (HLA) typing, for predisposition for cancer or for late onset diseases to the blond, blue-eyed six-foot athlete who serves their argumentative purposes so well. The discussion in the media of the new applications of PGD is replete with examples of tendentious labels all directed at pushing the discussion in a specific direction: 'designer babies', children as organ factories, the child as a 'medical product' or 'a commodity', a genetically 'custom-made' boy etc. The whole discussion would benefit from a more balanced and open approach in which the new applications are evaluated on their own merit.

We restrict our analysis to cases of 'parity for donation'. This term indicates that the practice not only involves the conception of a child but also its subsequent birth and its planned participation as a donor[2]. These cases should be distinguished from 'conception for donation' which involve situations where the embryo is created and later destroyed in order to harvest stem cells for therapy or where the fetus is electively aborted to obtain fetal tissue.

TRANSPLANTATION OF HEMATOPOIETIC STEM CELLS

For a number of diseases bone marrow transplantation is the only known cure. These disorders can be divided into three categories: immunodeficiency disorders, hematopoietic disorders and congenital metabolic disorders[3]. The success rate of transplantation varies significantly, depending on the disease type. The main complication associated with bone marrow transplantation is graft versus host disease, which is a major cause of morbidity and mortality after allogeneic transplants. The risk of graft versus host disease increases with HLA mismatch, the use of non-sibling familial donors, advanced donor age and donor-recipient sex mismatch[3]. In other words, a young same-sex HLA matched sibling is the best donor. Given the low number of children in a current family, the majority of patients do not have an HLA matched sibling or family member. The chance that a new sibling child is HLA matched with the affected child is 1 in 4. Although the birth of an HLA identical sibling does not guarantee the survival of the affected sibling, it is the best chance the child has.

The normal procedure if no matched sibling is available is to look for a matched unrelated donor in the national donor registries. The chance of finding a fairly compatible donor through these registries is around 75%. However, patients transplanted with marrow from a serologically matched unrelated donor suffer more often from post-transplant complications than those who are transplanted with marrow from an HLA-identical sibling[4]. The overall success rate of a transplant in a child with a sibling donor is substantially higher than of a transplant with alternative non-related donors. Even if a suitable unrelated donor could be found, parents might still prefer to conceive a related donor. However, they should be well aware of the risks and disadvantages of both IVF and PGD. During counseling, the probabilities and uncertainties associated with the PGD procedure and the transplantation should be stressed. Moreover, 'side issues' of the proposed treatment have to be considered beforehand. Parents should be urged to think about the disposition of the remaining embryos, about the possibility that few embryos are obtained and no matching embryo is found, about the possibility that no pregnancy follows and that the transplant fails or the sick child dies before the new child is born. This is a highly complex solution in which medico-technical, psychological and ethical dimensions must be combined. Prudence, extreme care and a thorough preparation are recommended.

ALTERNATIVE SOLUTIONS

From the moment that it became known that there is a considerable chance that siblings are suitable donors, parents started pregnancies in order to obtain a bone marrow donor for a sick child. As early as 1987 the conception of children to save older siblings was practiced[5]. The most famous case in the United States dates from 1990 and is known as the Ayala case. This middle-aged couple had a teenage daughter who was dying of cancer and needed a bone marrow transplant to survive. For some years an unrelated donor had been sought but none had been found. Neither the parents nor her brother proved to be compatible. Moreover, the father needed a reversal of a vasectomy performed 16 years earlier and the mother was already 42 years old. Against all odds (the final chance of success was estimated to be around 6%), they bore a daughter who was a suitable donor for her sister[6]. The transplantation was successful and the daughter married a few years later. A survey conducted by Kearney and Caplan revealed that the creation of babies specifically to serve as a bone marrow donor was not uncommon[2].

The possibility of determining the donor status of the fetus before birth generated the option of terminating the pregnancy if the fetus was unsuitable as a donor. In 1989 a debate was published on the question whether the selection of a fetus for bone marrow donation by means of prenatal diagnosis was morally acceptable[7,8]. Depending on the moral status attributed to the fetus, the ethical problems generated by this solution may be considered as very problematic.

Recently, the Nash case has caused a huge debate on the acceptability of the selection of embryos on HLA type by means of PGD[9]. This couple have a daughter with Fanconi anemia who was 6 years old at the time. Without a transplant she would have died in the next few years. The couple asked for PGD not only to test the embryos for Fanconi anemia but also to check their HLA type. HLA typing is a supplementary test in addition to the medically indicated test for the original disease. After four IVF cycles Mrs Nash became pregnant. After its birth, the umbilical cord cells of the donor child were used for transfusion of his elder sister and, as far as we know, everything is working out fine.

The evolution in the alternative solutions is completely determined by the increased knowledge and developing technology resulting in more refined and earlier applicable diagnostic tests. The first step is natural procreation in the hope of producing a suitable donor, the second step is a pregnancy followed by prenatal diagnosis and abortion if there is no match and finally, IVF followed by PGD to select the matching embryo(s). This evolution has brought progress on several levels: an increased possibility of obtaining a matching donor, shortening of the time and less burden on the woman.

THE PROS AND CONS OF PGD

PGD is a relatively new technique used to obtain genetic information about the embryos before implantation into the uterus[10]. The technique is used to identify affected embryos *in vitro* so that only unaffected embryos can be replaced. Originally it was offered to couples at high risk of transmitting genetic diseases as an alternative to conventional prenatal diagnosis possibly followed by therapeutic abortion. Later, the indications broadened. A major point of discussion at present is the use of PGD for aneuploidy screening. PGD has several advantages compared to natural procreation and prenatal selection. The first advantage is a consequence of the fact that *in vitro* fertilization (which necessarily precedes PGD) on average results in 10 to 12 embryos[11]. With several embryos to choose from, the probability that at least one embryo has the required HLA characteristic is high. Nevertheless, since in most cases these embryos also have to be analyzed for the disease mutation, the number of embryos which are both unaffected and a perfect HLA match may be small. In a recently reported case of 12 embryos only one embryo fulfilled both conditions[11]. This again speaks in favor of PGD as the solution. If the selection had to be carried out by means of prenatal diagnosis, there is a very high chance that the woman would have to undergo several terminations of pregnancy before success. Quite probably she would be forced to give up without a positive result.

Secondly, even if we count several IVF cycles before the woman gets pregnant, the average time needed to give birth to an HLA identical sibling will be much shorter than with any other method. For fast progressing diseases or diseases at an advanced stage, speed may be important. On the other hand, even with PGD one should reckon with a considerable delay. The practical development of a specific diagnostic multiplex polymerase chain reaction (PCR) may take several months. Add to this roughly three IVF cycles and 9 months' pregnancy and we have to take into account a total time period of approximately 1.5 years.

Finally, PGD may be easier on the couple (and especially on the woman), physically, psychologically and morally. Research indicates that women's attitudes towards PGD are largely influenced by previous experiences (for example prenatal diagnosis, abortion) and perception of genetic risk[12,13]. However, the claim made by opponents of PGD that the avoidance of abortion will lead to less stringent indications for selection (that is selection will take place for less serious diseases), is unsupported[14]. The necessity of undergoing one or more IVF cycles to obtain a suitable embryo and/ or to establish a pregnancy is arguably as high a barrier against trivial indications as termination of pregnancy. The assertion that PGD will be experienced as 'easy' by those who have to undertake this treatment is not corroborated by the available evidence[15].

Some people argue that the present application shows that the sliding down the slippery slope has already started. Originally PGD was developed to test embryos for serious genetic illnesses and to eliminate the risk of a child born with such a disease. In this case, however, there is nothing wrong with the embryos that are biopsied. The selection is made for a characteristic (that is the HLA genotype) that is useful to others. This determination of a feature of a future person, from which this person does not benefit himself, is morally problematic. Still, by extending the context in which the decision is framed, we reach a different perspective on the problem. We refer to the paragraph on the best interests and decision making within the family for a further analysis of this problem.

Would it make a difference if PGD for HLA typing is done as an additional test to PGD for mutation testing or if PGD is solely performed for HLA typing? There have already been requests for PGD for HLA matching as primary indication such as for leukemia[11]. In the latter cases, the effort of the IVF treatment is done solely for HLA matching. However, this difference does not seem relevant for acceptability. The risks and burden of an IVF treatment for the woman probably will not outweigh the benefit of saving her child's life.

THE CHILD AS AN INSTRUMENT

The main argument against this kind of request by the parents is the instrumentalization of the future child. The child becomes an instrument or medicine to cure another child[7]. To strengthen their position, the opponents invoke Kant's famous categorical imperative. The second formulation of the categorical imperative goes as follows: 'Act so that you treat humanity, whether in your own person or in that of another, always as an end and never as a means only'[16]. It is not always clear how it should be decided when someone is treated as a mere means and no longer as an end-in-himself[6]. It is generally agreed that using someone as a means is not unethical. An action should only be condemned when it treats a person *solely* as a means. When does an act instrumentalize a person? Parents frequently decide to have another child as a companion and a playmate for the previous one. Is the second child hereby treated as an instrument or not? These examples deserve serious scrutiny since such analysis might point at a possible explanation for our moral intuitions. When parents have a child as a companion for another child, this view does not preclude their intention to love the child and to raise it in the same way as the first child. When parents decide to have a child which can be used to cure another child, this reduces the child to a drug or a tissue sample. But then, why is the companion child not reduced to a toy or a pet? And how should we evaluate the replacement child? Suppose the transplantation is not successful and the affected child dies. The new child can then fill the void left by the dead child. Is wanting a child to replace another child less or more instrumentalizing than wanting a child that can also save the life of a sibling? When the parental decision is evaluated with this possible scenario in mind, it seems logical to decide to have another child which can possibly save the life of the existing child. It could even be argued that parents who want to have another child anyway, have an obligation to try this last possibility to save their sick child.

MOTIVES FOR PARENTHOOD

An important element in the discussion is the evaluation of the motives for parenthood. The opponents of HLA typing object to the inappropriate motive underlying the parents' wish for a child when they intend to use it as a donor. This objection is to a large extent connected with the conception of 'responsible parenthood'. This background theory is expressed in a number of principles. Two principles are important: good parents conceive a child for itself, and good parents accept the child as it comes[7]. Both principles also function in the rejection of interventions to select the sex and other characteristics of the future child[17]. The norm of unconditional acceptance of the child, however, is a dangerous argument in this context since any type of prenatal and preimplantation diagnosis (also mutation testing) 'presumes something less than unconditional acceptance of the child-to-be'[8].

Even if we accept that wanting a child for its own sake is the ideal, this does not imply that other motives are morally reprehensible. As Robertson rightly stated: 'While unqualified love and wanting children for their own sake may be the ideal, conceiving a child to be a bone marrow donor is not any worse or less altruistic than the myriad of other reasons for which children are sought'[18]. People have children in an attempt to save their marriage, to please their own parents, to confirm their image as man or woman, to help on the farm, to ensure caretakers in old age etc. A fair number of these reasons are parent-centered. Recently Heyd asserted that the decision to procreate 'is the only one in which the child is treated purely as a means (usually to the parents' satisfaction, wishes, and ideals)!'[19]. Although this statement seems too strong, it can be argued that to a certain extent all parents have children for themselves. This is no problem on the condition that this wish does not prevent loving and caring for the child as it is. The whole idea of wanting to morally evaluate the parents' motives is questionable and almost doomed to fail[20]. Given the presumption of reproductive liberty, parental motives are only judged when there is a risk of serious harm to future children[21].

Although it will be difficult to find a consensus on which motives for parenthood are acceptable, most people will agree on the statement that parents should respect their children as autonomous persons. This implies, to use Kant's categorical imperative again, that a person should never merely be treated as a means. Those who want to condemn the parental decision need to show that the intention to use a future child as a donor of hematopoietic stem cells is the only motive for having the child. It will be extremely difficult to demonstrate this. The main reason is that people usually have a multitude of motives for doing or choosing something. In general, we prefer to ignore this fact because it simplifies life if a person's act can be fully explained by one and only one clear motive. Most of the time we focus on those motives and reasons which allow us to make a quick moral evaluation of the act and/or person. The fact that some motives involve using the child is not unethical[18,22]. The claim that donation is the only parental motive cannot be established by looking at the parents' decision if one of the reasons falls away. The following non-ethical example can show this[23]. A woman decides to change jobs because at the new factory the salary is higher and she gets more days off. Suppose that the human resource manager changes his mind after the interview. He withdraws the original salary offer and proposes as much as she earns at present. The holiday benefit remains unchanged. If the woman alters her decision and stays at her current job, does this mean that the holidays did not influence her original decision? No. The change of mind shows at most that the days off alone were not sufficient to convince her.

Back to the selection problem. A couple state that they want another child because of reasons a and b. Suppose reason a is that they want to have a bone marrow donor for a sibling. Reason b is that they want another child as a companion for the first child. Imagine now that reason a no longer applies. This would be the case when prenatal diagnosis shows that the fetus is unsuitable as a donor or when after PGD no HLA matched embryos are found. The woman decides respectively to terminate the pregnancy or not to have any embryos transferred. If the parents abandon their parental project when they are informed that there is no possibility of tissue matching, this does not prove that they did not also truthfully want the child as a companion. It only shows that the companion motive was not in itself sufficient. Moreover, this situation does not show either that the donation motive is a singly sufficient reason. It is quite possible that both reasons together are only sufficient to persuade the parents to procreate.

The proof of an inappropriate attitude can only be made retrospectively. But even then we condemn the postnatal attitude of the parents regardless of the motive preceding the conception or birth. The clearest demonstration the parents could give of considering the child as a mere instrument is when they abandon it after taking the tissue. Robertson argues that even when the parents give up the child for adoption because it lacks the right tissue, this is still ethically defensible and falls within the range of the right to reproduce[18]. The child will presumably have a normal and reasonably happy life; the only difference with the normal situation is that it will be raised by adoptive parents. The child is not harmed (or need not be harmed) compared to the same child that would be raised by its genetic parents. Our indignation and repugnance of this parental decision is due to the fact that this act proves beyond doubt that the sole motive for having the child was its tissue. While it could be argued that the child is not harmed by being given up for adoption, it most certainly is wronged by being treated this way. The parents' behavior would be a blatant demonstration of disrespect. However, the discussion above is theoretical. Given the psycho-logic of the parental concern demonstrated by their efforts to save the sick child, it is highly unlikely that they will not treat the intended donor child as an equal to the existing child. The element of utility in the parents' decision to conceive does not cancel out their benevolent intentions to love and care for their child[24].

THE 'PRECEDING WISH' CONDITION

In the discussion of the different cases in the media, several people have stated that the request from the parents is only acceptable when they planned to have a child anyway. One of the physicians declared that he decided to do it, 'as long as the parents always intended to have a second baby and the tissue typing is just an add-on genetic test, rather than the *raison d'être* for the new child's life'[25]. The fact whether or not the family were intending to conceive another child is presented as morally relevant[6,26,27]. The existence or absence of such intention can be deduced from the statements the parents make about their desired family size or from some elements like the number of years since the last birth or a voluntary act like sterilization. The Ayala case, where the mother conceived 17 years after their last child and the husband had a vasectomy reversal, has all the indications of a new desire for a child.

The 'preceding wish' condition is rather peculiar. Suppose a couple want two children. After the second child is born, one of the parents is sterilized. A year later one of the children dies in a car accident. According to this condition, the parents cannot demand a reversal of the sterilization since they did not want another child before this happened. The child they wish for now is labeled a 'replacement' child. The same reasoning is applied to the HLA typing cases: the parents would not have the right to demand IVF combined with PGD if they had not wanted an additional child before they were informed of the illness of the existing child. But why should this new information about the possible death of a child not influence their family planning? Ironically, the only acceptable option open to the parents in this situation is to renounce further parenthood. If they decide not to conceive a possible bone marrow donor and the sick child dies, according to the same criterion, they should not be given assistance in having another child since it was not planned before this death.

The main purpose of the 'preceding wish' condition is to distinguish between the motives and reasons to conceive a child and the later use. The 'preceding wish' condition is based on the 'separation' principle[28]. This principle is applied in a multitude of situations in which the instrumental use of body material is envisioned. It states that there should be a complete separation between on the one hand the decision to conceive an embryo and the decision to abort a fetus and on the other hand the use that is made of the embryonic or fetal material. Owing to this principle it is requested that the decision to abort precedes the decision to donate fetal material for transplantation. The principle also underlies the arguments advanced by opponents of the intentional creation and destruction of embryos for research and for therapy. In a similar way, the demand that the parents should already have wanted or planned the future child before the need for a donor arose separates the motives for conception to some extent from the later use that is made of the material of the child. It wants to guarantee that the child will be respected regardless of its suitability as a donor. This condition seems all the more necessary since the increased control in obtaining a donor also reinforces the idea of 'production' and the conviction that the child is only conceived to use its cells[6].

The separation is never fully respected since the embryo is selected according to the HLA type. However, the main problem is that the separation principle starts from the premise that no benefit can ever justify conceiving and destroying or using an embryo or fetus. The principle builds heavily on a specific conception of the moral status of the embryo and fetus that is not shared by all. According to some the value created (or at least strived for), that is saving the life of a child, is sufficient to justify infringing the separation principle. The seriousness of the disease and the imminent death of the sick child should be taken into account to evaluate the parental decision. The real question is whether the critical health state of the sick child should be considered as a compelling reason for selecting the embryo(s). In normal circumstances the reason for eliminating affected embryos lies in the well-being of the potential future child. In HLA matching cases, the well-being of the existing sibling serves as the compelling reason.

The 'preceding wish' condition has a certain value because it indirectly demands that the parents should want and love the child that will be born. However, it is inappropriate because the postnatal attitude of the parents toward the child does not depend on the existence of a wish for a child before they were informed about the need for donor material. Luckily, the motivation (or absence thereof) to conceive does not fully determine the parental attitude toward the child that is born.

BEST INTERESTS AND DECISION MAKING WITHIN THE FAMILY

A major problem when incompetent persons are used as organ or tissue donors is the demonstration of their interests. This demonstration can be presented as an operational reformulation of the Kantian imperative that a person should always also be treated as an end. Being treated as a person can be identified with 'respecting his goals, desires, values etc.'. When it can be shown that the act serves an interest of the donor candidate, he or she is no longer treated solely as a means. This is not always easy or even feasible. In some cases the search and construction of interests seems rather far-fetched. In one case, to justify the harvesting of bone marrow from a severely mentally handicapped woman for the benefit of her younger sister, the court referred among other things to the possibility that the death of the patient would harm the donor because the health of the mother would be jeopardized, which in turn would result in less visiting of the donor by the mother[7]. This very much looks like a rationalization to explain what we feel that the final decision should be. This justification illustrates the general position taken in this debate. Since it is impossible to argue for medical benefits in case of organ or tissue donation, the focus is on psychological benefits. This usually proceeds by referring to the social situation and the psychologic benefits the donor has as a consequence of his relationship with the recipient and/or the other family members. The argument is based on a comparison of the expected quality of life of two possible children, child A who is HLA matched and child B who is unsuitable as a donor. If child A is born, its bone marrow or cord blood will be used to save the life of its older sibling. As a consequence, child A will grow up in an intact family. Child B, on the other hand, cannot donate and as a consequence will see its sibling die and will grow up in a family that is marked by the death of a child. From the point of view of the future child, it is beneficial to be able to save its sibling.

The idea underlying the classic interpretation is that we would be using the child if the net balance would disadvantage him or her. However, there are a large number of decisions in ordinary life taken by parents with more than one child where one child is harmed by a decision to benefit the other. They are vested with the authority to make such proxy decisions[29]. Suppose one child has special needs and has to go to a special school. If the parents decide to move in order to be closer to this special school, they harm the other sibling, who is losing his or her friends and familiar environment. This problem cannot be solved in such a way that both children benefit. The dilemma for parents is that they have to balance the interests of all their children. They judge that the sacrifice of the 'normal' sibling is justified by the gains of the needy child. If one child must suffer a small disadvantage in order to help his sibling a lot, the parents should take this decision. In fact, it can even be argued that not making this decision (not agreeing to the bone marrow donation of one sibling if there is a serious chance that the ill child can be saved) would be an unacceptable neglect of the existing child's interests. In conclusion, the donation can be justified by balancing the advantage of the recipient against the disadvantage for the donor in a close relationship.

However, the best interest standard is not the right model for donation of any tissue. Donations of body material are not justified by the benefits for the donor but by the promotion of the interests of the recipient. This basic element does not change in cases where the donor is incompetent. The incompetence forces us to consider other models to obtain the benefits while protecting the rights of the donor. The 'Good Samaritan' laws could serve as a useful model. These laws, although very controversial, are based on the idea that a person has a (non-elective) duty to help a person in need when he can do so at little or negligible cost to himself. In a loose analogy, it could be argued that an incompetent person (who by definition cannot choose to donate altruistically) can be 'volunteered' as a donor when the gains for the recipient are great compared to the costs for the donor. However, in order to prevent a self-serving interpretation of this balance, relatively strict standards and safety procedures have to be installed to protect the interests of incompetent persons.

VARIATIONS ON A THEME: RECIPIENTS AND GOALS

When HLA typing of future children is accepted, one should be prepared for future evolutions. It is possible to foresee new variations that will almost certainly present themselves. Two aspects should be considered: the goals of the selection and the recipients.

The postnatal test

It can reasonably be predicted that this technique will in time be proposed for disorders other than those which can be cured by hematopoietic stem cell transplantation. HLA matching would be useful in all those instances in which a member of the family needs an organ transplant. In one case a family conceived a child to provide a kidney for a child with chronic kidney failure[30]. In order to determine the acceptability of a motive for the selection of embryos, we suggest the 'postnatal' test. The 'postnatal' test states that it is ethically acceptable to have a child that can be used for a certain goal if it is acceptable to use an existing child for the same goal. This test is a necessary but not a sufficient condition for procreation. There are still the child's needs to be considered, for example the need to be loved and cared for in lasting, stable and warm personal relationships. If taking bone marrow from an infant is acceptable when the child exists (and came into existence independently of this decision), it is acceptable that one of the

61

motives for making the child is to have bone marrow. As Gerrand argued: 'Typically, to argue that an *intention to do X* is immoral, presupposes that *doing X* is immoral'[31]. So, the preconceptual intention to use a child as a bone marrow donor is not immoral if using an existing child as a donor is acceptable.

The postnatal test 'anticipates' the rights of the future child. No steps should be taken before conception that will infringe the rights of the future child once born. This raises the complex ethical question of using children and incompetent persons as donors of non-renewable organs. But if the parents have the decisional authority to volunteer an existing child as a bone marrow donor for a sibling, it is difficult to argue that they should not desire, as part of their motives for having a child, to make a child that can give bone marrow to a sibling. It follows from this criterion that parents cannot want a child for a certain reason if this means that something will be done to the child that is not allowed. If for instance taking a kidney from an infant to save its brother is unacceptable, it makes no sense to help parents to have a matching kidney donor.

When umbilical cord stem cells are used, there is no discomfort imposed on the donor. The risk associated with the collection of bone marrow (that is anesthesia and the possibility of complications, especially when the donor is very young) is completely eliminated. However, the sacrifice involved in bone marrow donation does 'not exceed the ordinary sacrifices family members make and expect from one another'[22]. There is general agreement that bone marrow donation represents a very low risk to the donor. The considerable benefit to the recipient in conjunction with the low risk imposed on the donor renders donorship (related and unrelated) for bone marrow ethically appropriate[32]. The more serious the harm (constituted by the pain, the risk of the intervention, the regenerability of the tissue etc.) the more difficult it becomes to justify the intervention.

When the recipient is not a sibling

Most authors who discuss these cases express their sympathy for the very difficult position in which the parents are placed. Even those who oppose parity for donation emphasize their understanding of the parents' wish to save their child. Views on parental responsibility and parental feelings justify at least a lenient attitude. However, how should we evaluate situations in which the recipient of the donor material is not the sibling but one of the parents or even another member of the family? Doctors are planning a similar procedure for thalassemia where the umbilical cord of the child could help cure the father[2,33]. Making a child to save one's own life certainly cannot expect as much goodwill from the population as making a child to save another child. Partially at least, the same reasoning can be applied as for donating to a sibling. The child that will be born HLA matched will be better off since it will have two healthy parents while its sibling who cannot serve as a donor will experience parental death or will grow up in a family with a chronically ill parent.

The argument that parents have the right and to a certain extent the obligation to do what they can to save their child is a major reason for accepting the application. As soon as self-interest enters the picture, the situation is evaluated differently. Is trying to save your own life an acceptable reason for creating and selecting embryos and bringing one of them into existence? The postnatal test does not exclude this application. If a child exists when the illness of the parent is discovered, it would be acceptable to use that child as a donor of bone marrow. The motive or reason the parents had for conceiving the child does not determine the relationship they intend to have with the child. Jecker argued that the motives underlying the start of a personal relationship decrease in importance when the relationship takes on a dynamic of its own[22]. The morally relevant point is not that parents have the right motive for conceiving the child but that they treat the child right and protect its best interests once it is born.

CONCLUSION

Conceiving a child to save another is a morally defensible decision on the condition that the operation that will be performed on the future child would be acceptable if the child already existed. The few instances in which parents have asked for medical intervention to obtain a compatible sibling strongly indicate that they really intend to love and care for the new child as they do for the sick child. The use or instrumentalization of that child does not demonstrate disrespect for his or her autonomy and intrinsic value.

REFERENCES

1. Mauron A, Thévoz J-M. Germ-line engineering: a few European voices. *J Med Phil* 1991;16:649–66
2. Kearney W, Caplan AL. Parity for the donation of bone marrow: ethical and policy considerations. In: Blank RH, Bonnicksen AL, eds. *Emerging Issues in Biomedical Policy*, Vol. 1, *Genetic and Reproductive Technologies*. New York: Columbia University Press, 1992:263–85
3. Wiley JM. Stem cell transplantation for the treatment of genetic disease. In: Kuller JA, Chescheir NC, Cefalo RC, eds. *Prenatal Diagnosis and Reproductive Genetics*. St. Louis, Missouri: Mosby, 1996:243–69
4. Tiercy JM, Bujan-Lose M, Chapuis B, *et al*. Bone marrow transplantation with unrelated donors: what is the probability of identifying an HLA-A/B/Cw/DRB1/B3/DQB1-matched donor? *Bone Marrow Transpl* 2000;26:437–41
5. Burgio GR, Nespoli L, Forta F. Programming of bone marrow donor for a leukaemic sibling. *Lancet* 1987;339:1484–5

6. Drebushenko DW. Creating children to save siblings' lives: a case study for Kantian ethics. In: Humber J, Almeder R, eds. *Bioethics and the Fetus.* Totowa, New Jersey: Humana Press, 1991:89–101

7. Clark RD, Fletcher J, Petersen G. Conceiving a fetus for bone marrow donation: an ethical problem in prenatal diagnosis. *Prenat Diagn* 1989;9:329–34

8. Fost N. Guiding principles for prenatal diagnosis. *Prenat Diagn* 1989;9:335–7

9. Verlinsky Y, Rechitsky S, Schoolcraft W, Strom C, Kuliev A. Designer babies – are they a reality yet? Case report: simultaneous preimplantation genetic diagnosis for Fanconi anaemia and HLA typing for cord blood transplantation. *Reprod Bio Med* 2000;1:31

10. Handyside AH, Kontogianni EH, Hardy K, Winston RM. Pregnancies after biopsied human preimplantation embryos sexed for Y-specific DNA amplification. *Nature* 1990;344:768–70

11. International Working Group on Preimplantation Genetics. Tenth anniversary of preimplantation genetic diagnosis. *J Assoc Reprod Gen* 2001;18:64–70

12. Miedzybrodzka Z, Templeton A, Dean J, Haites N, Mollison J, Smith N. Preimplantation diagnosis or chorionic villus biopsy? Women's attitudes and preferences. *Hum Reprod* 1993;8:2192–6

13. Palomba ML, Monni G, Lai R, Cau G, Olla G, Cao A. Psychological implications and acceptability of preimplantation diagnosis. *Hum Reprod* 1994;9: 360–2

14. King DS. Preimplantation genetic diagnosis and the 'new' genetics. *J Med Ethics* 1999;25:176–82

15. Lavery SA, Aurell R, Turner C, Trew G, Margara R, Winston RML. Patients' perspectives of preimplantation genetic diagnosis and its psychological impact. *Hum Reprod* 2000;15, (Abst)1:94

16. Kant I. *Foundations of the Metaphysics of Morals.* New York: MacMillan, 1959

17. Pennings G. Family balancing as a morally acceptable application of sex selection. *Hum Reprod* 1996;11:2339–45

18. Robertson JA. *Children of Choice: Freedom and the New Reproductive Technologies.* Princeton, New Jersey: Princeton University Press, 1994

19. Heyd D. *Genethics: Moral Issues in the Creation Of People.* Berkeley: University of California Press, 1992

20. Zucker A. Baby marrow: ethicists and privacy. *J Med Ethics* 1992;18:125–7,141

21. Kahn J. Making lives to save lives. *J Androl* 2001;22:191

22. Jecker NS. Conceiving a child to save a child: reproductive and filial ethics. *J Clin Ethics* 1990;1:99–103

23. Honoré T. Necessary and sufficient conditions in tort law. In: Owen DG, ed. *Philosophical Foundations of Tort Law.* Oxford: Clarendon Press, 1995:363–85

24. Sharpe VA. To what extent should we think of our intimates as "persons"? Commentary on *Conceiving a Child. J Clin Ethics* 1990;1:103–7

25. Boyce N. Designing a dilemma. *New Scientist*, December 11, 1999:18–19

26. De Wert G. Erfelijkheidsonderzoek en ethiek: een gordiaanse knoop. *Wijsg Perspect* 2000;40:150–6

27. Edwards RG. A well-taken opportunity for double blessing. *Reprod Bio Med* 2000;1:31–3

28. Pennings G. Ethical issues in the use of human embryonic stem (ES) cells. In: *Syllabus Pre-congress Course Ethics and Law*. Presented at the *17th Annual Meeting ESHRE, Lausanne, Switzerland*, 1 July 2001:13–18

29. Ross LF. Justice for children: the child as organ donor. *Bioethics* 1994;8: 105–26

30. Norton VG. Unnatural selection: nontherapeutic preimplantation genetic screening and proposed regulation. *UCLA Law Rev* 1994;41:1581–650

31. Gerrand N. Creating embryos for research. *J Appl Phil* 1993;10:175–87

32. Ethics Committee of the United Network for Organ Sharing (UNOS). Principles of organ and tissue allocation and donation by living donors. *Transplant Proc* 1992;24:2226–37

33. Browne A, McKie R. We'll have that one – it's perfect. *The Guardian*, October 8, 2000

5

Multiple pregnancies and our responsibility to ART children

J. Cohen

INTRODUCTION

The marked increase in multiple births attributable to assisted conception techniques is well documented. Concern has been expressed about the psychological and social effects of these techniques on the potential children and their parents. The aim of this chapter is to discuss the moral responsibility of clinicians and biologists to the children born from an assisted reproductive technology (ART) multiple pregnancy.

ASSISTED CONCEPTION AND MULTIPLE PREGNANCIES

In the developed countries around 1% of babies born per year result from *in vitro* fertilization (IVF) and other ART procedures. International registries indicate a high incidence of multiple pregnancies. In a population-based study in Denmark[1], the national incidence of multiple pregnancies increased 1.7-fold during 1980 to 1994, the increase coming primarily in 1989–94 and almost exclusively in primiparous women aged 30 years, for whom the adjusted proportion based twinning rate increased 2.7-fold and the triplet rate 9.1-fold. During 1989–94 the adjusted yearly increase in multiple pregnancies for these women was 19%. The proportion of multiple births among those infants who died – in primiparous women of 30 years – increased from 11.5% to 26.9% during the study period. The authors concluded that the introduction of new treatments to enhance fertility (not all of them concerning IVF) has probably caused these changes.

According to the French National Register on *In Vitro* Fertilization (FIVNAT)[2] from 1986 to 1993 in France the birth rate of twins after IVF was 23.5% and the rate of triplets or more babies was 3.75%. If we consider the rate of triplets or more before embryo reduction, the rates were 7.3% at conception, 6.5% before reduction and 3.8% at birth[1]. In 2000 FIVNAT[3] published the outcome of pregnancies from IVF and intracytoplasmic sperm injection (ICSI) obtained between 1995 and 1998. The birth rates of twins were 26.1% (IVF) and 24.2% (ICSI). The rates for triplets were, respectively, 1.5% and 1.6%. There was only one quadruplet in each group. The embryo reduction rate was 2.8% for IVF and 2.3% for ICSI.

These figures show that progress has been made in France as regards the rates of multiple births owing to the reduction in the number of embryos transferred. But the problem remains important in many countries, and even in France the total of triplet births and embryo reductions shows that triplets constitute at least 4.3% of assisted pregnancies. Embryo reduction also has its specific physiologic and psychologic complications.

The main risk in multiple pregnancy stems from the very high rate of preterm delivery. In addition, low birth weight and intrauterine growth retardation are more frequent in twins and higher multiple-gestation fetuses, both resulting in high neonatal and infant mortality rates. Mortality *in utero* increases from 6.2% to 30.2% from singleton to triplets, and total neonatal mortality from 6% to 32.9% (FIVNAT)[2].

In a review of 12 publications Berkowitz and associates[4] noted 707 triplet pregnancies with 90% of deliveries before 37 weeks, 24% of deliveries before 32 weeks and 8% of deliveries before 28 weeks. Although the IQ of the children is normal and the majority are free of major handicaps, there is an increased incidence of developmental disability, cerebral palsy, mental retardation, sensory impairment, language delays, learning disability and attention and behavioral problems in children resulting from multiple pregnancies. Also the life of the couple who experience a high-order multiple pregnancy is drastically changed for years to come.

From a purely financial and utilitarian point of view, it is obvious to anyone who calculates cost that prevention of preterm deliveries in multiple pregnancies is highly cost effective. Multiple pregnancies in IVF do not seem to differ in terms of obstetric and perinatal outcomes from spontaneous multiple pregnancies or pregnancies obtained after ovarian stimulation but without IVF-embryo transfer (ET). Olivennes and colleagues[5] in a retrospective analysis showed that in the IVF-ET group prematurity rate (38.9%), small for gestation age (18%) and perinatal mortality (3.47%) were not statistically different from a stimulation group without IVF (45.1%, 23.2% and 3.05%, respectively) and a spontaneous group (39.6%, 22.7% and 4.27%, respectively). Craandjik[6] compared 224 spontaneously achieved twin pregnancies, 22 achieved by ovarian stimulation and 52 by IVF. Fetal growth retardation was observed in 17.4%, 18% and 21.2%, respectively and preterm delivery in 33.3%, 22.7% and 51.9%, respectively. Significant differences were not found.

Nevertheless, a reduction in the proportion of multiple pregnancies, including twin gestation, should be a goal for IVF-ET teams.

Controlled ovarian stimulation (COS) is also a very significant risk factor for multiple pregnancies. In France in 1993, 40% of triplets were born after IVF, 35% after ovulation induction and 25% were spontaneous. Norwitz[7] indicated that ovulation induction accounted for 10–69% of triplets, ART for 24–30% and 7–18% were spontaneous. There are little data available regarding multiparity after COS.

PSYCHOSOCIAL DILEMMAS CONCERNING CHILDREN BORN FROM MULTIPLE PREGNANCIES

Multiple births present particular problems to the parents, as indicated by MacWhinnie's study[8]. Studies of triplet families indicate that the risk of family disruption is high, with an incidence in the range from 1 in 4 to 1 in 3 and the risk to the babies (prematurity and its complications, such as cerebral hemorrhage or chronic lung disease) is important. Parental disruption, of course, has concomitant effects on the children.

Botting and coworkers[9] listed the following aspects that parents of triplets and 'higher-order' multiple-birth children have to deal with:

(1)   Feeding premature babies; they are smaller and feed more slowly than full-term babies.

(2)   Changing clothes and nappies, and incessant washing and drying.

(3)   Sleep can become a major problem, for example one crying baby wakes the other two.

(4)   Getting out of the house with three babies involves getting them all ready at the same time. Visits to the clinic and doctor become a major expedition. Even with a car available to the parent, at least one other adult is needed.

(5)   Public transport is much too daunting, if not impossible.

(6)   Lack of sleep and exhaustion become major concerns.

The general result is that visits to friends cease as other mothers with young children are unwilling to have three extra to stay over, while baby-sitting to allow parents to go out on their own is a major problem. Finance is also a problem, particularly when the family budget had relied on the mother's earnings. Fathers have to take on extra hours at work to replace the reduced income and meet the increased costs; as a result they are less available to help with the children.

This analysis takes no account of the dramatic increase in hospital charges associated with multiple births. Callahan and colleagues have shown that the charges in 1991 were $9845 for a singleton, $37 947 for twins and $109 765 for triplets in the USA[10].

Garel and coworkers studied 11 mothers of triplets[11,12]. After 7 years three of the mothers were still suffering from depressive symptoms. The mothers' psychological distress and the quality of their relationship with their children remained serious preoccupations in two of the families. The correlation between depression in mothers and the well-being of their children has been established by numerous research studies. In a review of these, Rutter and colleagues[13] conclude that maternal depression is a psychologic risk factor for the children. while Bryan and coworkers state that there is a risk of nonaccidental injuries for these children[14]. Furthermore Tanimura and associates found in a nationwide survey in Japan that 10% of child abuse victims were products of multiple births[15]. This represents almost ten times the incidence in the population as a whole. A smaller study in the USA arrived at a similar general conclusion[16].

DISCUSSION

The desire for a child is at the center of different interests: the individual, society, our symbolic representation and our actual being. Many women – but fewer men – are driven by this impulse towards maternity (or paternity), obeying laws of an unconscious nature. For several decades and in particular since the spread of treatments for sterility and infertility, the notion of a 'right to a child' has appeared. Infertile couples have obtained recognition of their suffering and in many countries this right of atonement for the misfortune they have been enduring has meant that insurance companies and health services cover the expenses of infertility treatments. At the same time since efficient and well tolerated contraception has been fully accepted, women have acquired the possibility (asserted as a right) to have or not to have a child whenever it is most appropriate in their lives. In a great number of countries this privilege has led to the possibility of voluntary and legal interruption of pregnancy. Does not this new phenomenon of 'A child if I want one and when I want one', this new possibility to satisfy the yearning of adults for children, lead to instrumentalization of the child or the 'children seen as objects'? So, little by little, in Western societies a child with a new status emerges. He/she is exceptional, more valued and also more yearned for when he/she comes into the world.

Oddly enough at a time when everyone is preoccupied by the suffering of couples, the rights of women and the means to purvey infertility treatments, the effects of technical or social mutations on the child-to-be are rarely tackled. These effects are almost never seen on the day the child is born, unless there is a major handicap. They appear after a few years and will be recognized and studied only if a greater number of individuals affected express their situation and claim recognition. Decades have been necessary to recognize that Rhesus negative baby girls had been Rhesus positive immunized by hemotherapy that was so widespread in the 1930s. Later in the century the quest for identity by adopted abandoned children or children born thanks to gamete donation reminds us that a child who has been so much yearned for can one day itself turn into one who yearns.

But what is new is the major part played by doctors and biologists in the 'creation' or 'making' of these children. Many infertile couples state strongly that the doctor played the part of a 'surrogate parent', thus stressing the very special part of the technical aid supplied to the couple. Without the doctor there would not be a child. He/she is in a way a 'godparent' to the child-in-making – even if in this situation he/she stands for medicine at large. To mention godparent implies responsibility toward the godchild. At present this responsibility is only indicated through the general principle: the actors in assisted procreation must take into account in advance the welfare of the child to be and this is seldom done apart from in the UK, for it is extremely difficult to find the proper means.

A different matter is the problem of the quality of life of the child in his teens or when he/she reaches adulthood.

Would a child with a psychological or physical handicap directly linked to ART not be entitled to sue those responsible for his existence and present state? Of course the first to be accountable might be the parents, whose decision initiated the process. They might therefore assert that they were ignorant of the effects of the technique, but doctors and biologists will not be able to do the same. They bear the moral responsibility for having practiced a treatment or a technique of whose possible risks they were aware … or had not double-checked the absence of ill-fated consequences. This can apply in particular to the problem of multiple pregnancies after infertility treatment. Couples treated without success, those losing a child during the pregnancy, or those whose married life disintegrated because of too many children will challenge our responsibility in the near future. But handicapped children, their brothers and sisters, and those whose parents separated because of their very existence, will be entitled to question the responsibility of doctors in their suffering. The personal responsibility of doctors will be addressed as different attitudes towards the prevention or resolution of multiple pregnancies prevail. Awareness of our responsibilities must lead to three types of medical action.

Prevention

We know it is possible to avoid pregnancies of a rank superior to two by transferring only one embryo in auspicious cases or by transferring two embryos at most. In these two cases there would be cryopreservation of the remaining embryos.

The ideal situation would be to be able to detect, before transfer, the perilous cases in order to transfer more than two embryos only in the few cases where the risk is small. However this is not yet possible and therefore it may lead to multiple pregnancies. The assertion that informed parents have chosen the transfer of several embryos is morally challengeable as those prospective parents are in such a state of anguish and impatience that their judgment is being impaired. Even if parents are willing to take a chance the doctor does not have the moral right to accept. He morally represents the child who has no possibility to choose a risk for himself or herself.

Moreover it has recently been shown that the strategy of transferring a limited number of embryos does not damage the chances of the potential parents of having a child when there remain frozen embryos in reserve.

Embryo reduction

Embryo reduction is a technique that cannot be morally condemned by those who accept abortion. It can be criticized by those who feel that the embryo is already a human being by all means, but these must be fully aware of the risks and consequences of multiple pregnancies before any assisted medical procreation. Ethically there is no reason to deny embryo reduction in itself. However we know there is a risk of losing all the embryos (5 to 10% according to different authors) and it becomes morally absurd to suppress pregnancies which were so painful to obtain. Embryo reduction is a solution doctors may offer in the case of a multiple pregnancy if it is not presented as an innocuous way of dealing with multiple embryo transfer and the couple (or the wife) have been warned of the risk of total pregnancy loss or any other complication when this technique is used.

Social measures

Social measures should be introduced in favor of parents of children born of multiple pregnancies. We know some multiple pregnancies may occur spontaneously and in spite of all precautions. The state, as well as insurance companies, plays a part in subsidizing fertility treatment. The pharmaceutical industry makes huge profits thanks to the prescription of these treatments. It is therefore fair (and justified) that society seeks to compensate a handicap that it helped create: allocation of sufficient maternal aid, social and psychological support for these couples who all say how unprepared they were to face the enormous difficulties encountered when raising and educating several children of the same age.

Doctors must draw the attention of the public as well as that of government establishments to the urgency and importance of such measures. They must help benevolent associations who work in this field and give them the means to state their case publicly. Another measure for doctors and centers would be to express the effectiveness of IVF in terms of singleton births. Multiple pregnancies (including twins) should be reported separately as complications of treatment. This would avoid misleading the public, and promote the right message by proper information.

As we have seen we practitioners have a major responsibility. We cannot dodge it by pleading ignorance. For future parents as well as future children we must be able to evaluate the risks of new techniques and start a treatment only once the well-being of the future child has been ensured or at least iatrogenic complications of a magnitude we cannot ignore avoided.

Finally, the means to safety should be debated: are professional codes of practice sufficient or do we need the strong arm of the law? In other words, in a matter which arguably is also a matter of public health as well as personal responsibility of the practitioner towards future parents and their child, does society decide that it is necessary to limit the medical profession's autonomy by legislation rather than to continue the ideal relation of trust between the carer and the individual patient and society? Only evidence-based medicine can help us to decide, like that of the European Society for Human Reproduction and Embryology group which enables analysis of the rate of multiple pregnancies in different European countries. This, taken with the American Society for Reproductive Medicine figures, may help or force a decision unless the profession decides to act in what is currently one of the main complications of ART techniques.

REFERENCES

1. Westegaard T, Wohlfahrt J, Bolton V, *et al.* Population based study of rates of multiple pregnancies in Denmark. *Br Med J* 1997;314:775–9
2. FIVNAT grossesses multiples. *Contrac Fertil Sex* 1995;23:494–7
3. FIVNAT, Bilan de l'année 1999. J. de Mouzon. INSERM U292. Kremlin Bicêtre, France
4. Berkowitz RL, Lynch L, Stone J, Alvarez M. The current status of multifetal pregnancy reduction. *Am J Obstet Gynecol* 1996;174:1265–72
5. Olivennes M, Kadher P, *et al.* Perinatal outcome of twin pregnancies after IVF. *Fertil Steril* 1996;66:105–9
6. Graandjik M. The influence of assisted procreation on the perinatal outcome of twin pregnancies. *Hum Reprod* 1996;11:40
7. Norwitz ER. Multiple pregnancy: trends, past, present and future. *Infertil Reprod Clin North Am* 1998;9:351–69
8. MacWhinnie A. Families from assisted conception: ethical and psychological issues. *Hum Fertil* 2000;3:13–19
9. Botting BJ, MacFarlane AJ, Price FV. Three, four and more: a study of triplets and higher order births. London: Her Majesty's Stationery Office
10. Callahan TL, Hall JE, Ettner SL, Christiansen CL, Greene MF, Crowley WF Jr. The economic impact of multiple-gestation pregnancies and the contribution of assisted-reproduction techniques to their incidence. *N Engl J Med* 1994;331:244–9
11. Garel M, Salobir C, Blondel B. Assessment at 4 years of the psychological consequences of having triplets. *Fertil Steril* 1997;8:1162–5
12. Garel M, Salobir C, Lelong N, Blondel B. Les mères de triplés et leurs enfants (in French). *Gynecol Obstet Fertil* 2000;28:792–7

13. Rutter M, Bolton P, Harrington R, *et al*. Genetic factors in child psychiatric disorders. *J Child Psychol Psychiatr* 1990;31:3–37
14. Bryan EM, Denton J, Hallett F. *Facts about Multiple Births. Guidelines for Professionals*. London: Multiple Births Foundation
15. Tanimura M, Matsui I, Kobayashi N. Child abuse of one of a pair of twins in Japan. *Lancet* 1990;336:1298–9
16. Groothuis JR, Attemeier WA, Robarge JP, *et al*. Increased child abuse in families with twins. *Pediatrics* 1982;70:769–73

6

Gamete donation: secrets and anonymity

J. Tizzard

INTRODUCTION

Donor insemination (DI) has been practiced for nearly 100 years, making it the oldest form of assisted conception in humans. But despite its lengthy service, DI has only relatively recently emerged from a shadow of secrecy and shame[1]. Until recently, doctors advised couples to keep the donation a secret from family and friends – and the resulting child – because no-one needed to know. The female partner got pregnant and delivered the baby as normal, so the illusion that the male partner was also the genetic father could be preserved. The anonymity of the sperm donor has been the preferred system since DI was first offered as a clinical service. Even as late as 1960, when a British report on artificial insemination by donor was published, non-anonymous donation was thought to attract 'the abnormal and the unbalanced'[2]. Times have changed. Over the past few years debate about the merits of anonymous and known gamete donation has raged in professional and public arenas. Some countries maintain a system of anonymous donation, others have moved to known donation, while a handful offer a choice between both systems. The aim of this essay is to assess those systems of service provision and suggest a way forward for policy making in the area.

SECRETS IN GAMETE DONATION

Gamete donor anonymity might still be the norm in most countries offering treatment. But do parents tell their child how they were conceived, despite the lack of identifying information about the donor? Research carried out on families born of different assisted conception techniques shows that parents of children born of donated gametes are less likely to tell their child how they were conceived than parents of children born of IVF without donated gametes. In one study 50% of IVF parents had told their child how they were conceived by the time they were 12 years old. By contrast, only 9% of DI parents had told their child[3].

While most medical practitioners and counselors now advise patients seeking donor conception treatment to be open with their children, it seems that parents tend not to heed that advice. Why is this? We do not know for sure, but parents in studies express a number of different reasons for not telling: they intend to tell, but never find the right time to do it; they are concerned that the child might love the father (in the case of DI) less; or they find it too difficult to explain donor conception to a young child, then consider it too late when the child is old enough to understand the technicalities. Some parents feel that telling their child about their conception, when anonymity means they will never meet the donor, would be pointless or even cruel[4]. A smaller number of parents, for cultural or religious reasons, feel completely unable to reveal the circumstances of their child's conception for fear of being ostracized.

Given the small number of studies carried out on donor conception parents, we still know relatively little about why parents choose to tell or not to tell their children. But is donor anonymity a significant factor? Wincott and Hedgley believe it is. 'This denial [of identifying information about the donor] creates a climate where secrecy about origins can flourish, which can be very damaging'[5].

It seems that some parents decide not to tell because of donor anonymity. But it might also be the case that they never intended to tell and that anonymity protects this secret. The opposite relationship between anonymity and secrecy might equally be true: parents could tell their children, safe in the knowledge that a donor will never be revealed to run the risk of disrupting family relations. If this were true, the low rate of telling in donor conception families would have more to do with the other factors mentioned above. A final possible explanation for not telling is that parents fear that anonymity laws will be changed retrospectively and they therefore fear the donor getting in contact at a later date. If they had more faith in law-makers, they might tell their child the truth.

Unfortunately, much of the association between secrecy and anonymity – if indeed there is one – is currently based upon guesswork. If a relationship exists, it is probably a complex one and, until further studies are carried out, we do not fully understand it.

ANONYMOUS AND KNOWN DONATION

Most countries which offer donor conception treatments do so through an anonymous system, although there is an increasing variety in approaches[6]. Some countries have a system of collecting non-identifying information about the donor which the offspring can access at a particular age (usually at legal maturity). In the United Kingdom, since legislation came into force in 1991, all clinics recruiting egg, sperm and embryo donors must collect a medical and family history of the donor, they must carry out appropriate carrier screening for genetic diseases and they must screen the gametes for common viruses such as HIV. Donors also have the opportunity to record other information such as their interests. These records, containing non-identifying information about the donor, may be available for view by the offspring at the age of 18[7].

In some countries where anonymous donation is the norm, a method of recruiting known donors is sometimes used. Prospective parents are asked to recruit their own donor from friends or family. The donor gametes are then put into a 'pool', whereby they are offered to another couple, while those who recruited the donor go to the top of the waiting-list and receive gametes from another donor in the pool who is unknown to them. This is often a popular way of recruiting egg donors.

Other countries occupy a kind of middle ground by offering a 'double track' system wherein the prospective parents can choose between anonymous and known donation[8]. The Netherlands currently offers this choice, although it is designed as a transition system between anonymous and known donation. A number of clinics in California in the United States offer an 'identity release' service, providing prospective parents with an alternative to anonymous donation services elsewhere in the country.

A small number of legislatures, such as Austria, Sweden and the state of Victoria, Australia, have moved to allow offspring access to identifying information about the donor. In 1992 Austria passed legislation which gives donor offspring the right, at the age of 14, to learn the identity of the donor. The Swedish law, enacted in 1985, states that children born of donor insemination have the right, at maturity, to access identifying information about the donor. But the right is not strong. Because no one other than the parents can inform the child, the right to know the identity of one's genetic father is contingent upon the child's knowing that they were born of donor conception treatment. The laws in Austria and Sweden apply only to children born of donor insemination, since egg donation is outlawed in both countries.

A QUESTION OF RIGHTS?

The interests of the three parties to donor assisted conception – donors, parents and offspring – are often discussed in terms of rights. How do we characterize those rights? There are a number of legal rights, at national, continental and international levels, which have been associated with the different parties involved in donor assisted conception.

Donors/gamete providers

National common law or statute often provides a basic protection of the donor's confidentiality. Whatever information is released to the prospective parents and to the future child, is done so with the consent of the donor. However, the donor has a duty not to withhold relevant family or medical information. Explicit withholding of such information would mean that they were not accepted onto a gamete donation program. In the United Kingdom, if a donor knowingly (but not explicitly) withholds relevant family or medical information and the resulting child is born disabled as a direct result, the child has a legal claim of damages[9]. Under the European Convention on Human Rights (ECHR) the donor also has a right to 'private and family life'[10]. 'Private life' includes the right to control personal information and to make one's own treatment decisions. But a right to 'family life' does not extend to children born as a result of his or her donation.

Recipients/prospective parents

Similar rights of confidentiality and rights under the ECHR apply to the prospective parents as they do to gamete donors. But the 'right to private and family life' is not a positive right and so would probably not apply to access to fertility treatment. However, it might also mean that no party outside the family could legitimately intervene to tell a child of its donor status. Article 12 of the convention provides a 'right to marry and found a family', though a recent case in the UK suggests that this does not mean a right to conceive a child under any circumstances[11].

Offspring/children

If a donor has no right to family life with the child which results from the donation, it is unlikely that the child has a right to family life with the donor, since there is no mention of genetic ties in family life. Genetics is also missing from the relevant articles of the United Nations Convention on the Rights of the Child, which is often used to justify abolition of donor anonymity[12]. The convention talks of a 'right to know one's parents' and a 'right of the child to preserve his or her identity'[12]. These articles were drawn up to protect children who are forcibly removed from their parents, presumably regardless of whether they are genetically related or not.

Many of these legal mechanisms remain untested in the courts, so it is unclear at this stage exactly how to interpret them. It seems that there is a right to know one's parents, but is it correct to view a gamete donor as a parent? One sperm donor explained his motivation: 'I donated sperm to assist another couple become parents of "their child". I did not donate sperm to become a father again'[5]. However, one journalist has said of donor insemination: 'what seems extraordinary is that men were ever encouraged to become fathers so lightly'[13]. Egg and sperm donors cannot be regarded as parents in any meaningful sense. Parenting is usually understood to mean caring for children, bringing them up and being responsible for their transition into adulthood. Gamete donors provide none of these important functions of parenting. Even in countries where some right to know one's genetic parents has been accorded to people born of gamete donation, the right seems to be inconsistently applied. A recent Swedish study shows that of 80% of the people who had become DI parents since 1985, just 52% had told or intended to tell their children about their donor status[14]. Swedish donor conception children might have a legal right to know their donor's identity, but it is a right which is currently unenforced.

Any right we might have to know our genetic parents is also commonly flouted elsewhere in cases of marital infidelity, when a person wrongly assumes that his or her social father is also the genetic father (estimated to be as high as one in seven people). A number of commentators have challenged the use of this analogy, arguing that such family deceit sets a poor example for policy making[12]. But the example of wrongly assumed paternity is not meant as a justification for, or an encouragement of, parents deceiving their children. Nor is it meant as a basis on which to formulate policy. It is simply to demonstrate that if a right to know one's genetic parents exists, it is a right that is commonly flouted – much more often in natural conception than in donor conception. The fact that many children conceived without medical assistance – those conceived after a one-night stand perhaps – do not know the identity of their genetic father weakens the case that a right to know one's genetic parents exists. Given that records are kept nowadays about gamete donors, these children probably know less about their genetic father than children born of donor insemination do.

Adoptive children

Adoption is often likened to donor assisted conception in respect of secrecy and anonymity. Golombok has rejected the view that because adopted children and children born of gamete donation lack a genetic link with one or both parents, their psychologic experiences have much in common.

> 'The child [born of donor insemination] does have a genetic relationship with one parent, the mother. The child is born to the mother, and the child has not been given up by the biological parents. In all of these ways, donor insemination families are more like natural families than adoptive ones'[4].

This also applies to egg donation where, although the mother is not genetically related, she carries the pregnancy. It could be argued that because adopted children are able to trace their birth parents at the age of maturity, they do have and can exercise a right to know their genetic parents. But is this true? From Golombok's description of an adopted child's experience, there is an important distinction: adopted children were born to their genetic mother and given up by her for adoption as a baby or as a child. As such, that child had a – possibly fleeting – relationship with their genetic mother that was broken in some way. Gamete donors do not have a similar relationship with the child which results from their donation, since it could not be argued that giving up eggs, sperm or embryos is at all comparable to giving up a baby or child. As such, adopted children seem to have a right to know the identity of their birth mother, rather than their genetic mother, even though this is the same person. One other factor is that adopted children do not always seek their genetic parents, and when they do they tend to seek the birth mother only. This suggests again that gestation and birth are the bonding factors, rather than a genetic tie[15].

THE UK HUMAN RIGHTS ACT

It is often suggested that children born of anonymous donor conception are denied their most basic human rights. 'They are the only group in this country who don't have the right in law to trace their genetic parents – a fundamental violation of their human rights'[5]. We have already reviewed the relevant articles of the European Convention on Human Rights and how they might be applied to donor assisted conception. But what about domestic law?

According to reports in British publications, two adults born of donor insemination, Adam Rose and his sister Joanna, plan to challenge the ban on the release of identifying information about donors to the offspring. The case, to be fought by the civil liberties organization Liberty, on behalf of the Rose siblings and a number of donor offspring adults, will challenge the current law under the UK Human Rights Act 1998, which incorporated the European Convention on Human Rights into UK law in October 2000[16]. Some months after the announcement, it remains unclear exactly what the legal argument of this claim will be and when – and if – it will come to court.

THE WELFARE OF THE CHILD

Over the past decade the idea that the welfare of children born of assisted conception techniques ought to be considered has gained in popularity. Although this idea is often poorly defined and inconsistently applied[17], it has become one of the main factors for deciding whether or not treatment is ethically acceptable. So, even if rights are not being contravened by anonymous donation, does it undermine a child's welfare? Some philosophers have argued that assisted conception techniques always promote the welfare of children. Because these techniques are designed to bring about the birth of children, and it is usually thought that being alive is a good thing (and certainly preferable to the alternatives), child welfare is never undermined, unless that child's life is so compromised as to make it not worth living[18]. In short, one can never be harmed by being born. This is obviously true, but a more precise question might illuminate our discussion of known and anonymous gamete donation. Is the welfare of a child born of anonymous donation so compromised that we ought not to offer it at all, even as an option alongside known donation?

Are children or adults born of gamete donation harmed by not knowing about the donation? Unfortunately, we do not really know. The Golombok studies (where most parents have not told their offspring) seem to suggest that such secret keeping is not harmful to the child. But the children have been seen only up to the age of 12. Turner's and Coyle's study of adults born of gamete donation show that family secrets can be damaging.

> 'A consistent finding within the study was the negative and ongoing effects of withholding secrets and the knowledge that "things were not quite right"... Although disclosure in adulthood was reported as shocking, participants reported that "knowing" their status initiated a re-evaluation and resolution of previously unanswered, unresolved family experiences' [19].

The 16 participants in this study obviously know about their donor status – something which has clearly had a profound impact upon them – so their reliability as objective witnesses is questionable. While the study gives valuable insights into the impact of finding out the truth, it is difficult to draw any conclusions from it about whether children really do know when an important secret is being kept.

What about anonymity? Do offspring who know want to trace the donor? Turner's and Coyle's study suggests that they do. All of the participants had made some initial enquiries about searching for their donors and all expressed a sense of loss at not being able to know who their donors were[19]. However, the findings should be seen in the context of a small, qualitative study in which the participants discovered how they were conceived in a number of different circumstances. The authors recognize the problems of recruiting participants through support networks, because they may be more likely to need to talk and resolve identity issues. As a result these people might be more likely to desire identifying information about the donor.

One survey of people born through donor insemination, published in a support group newsletter, showed that a large majority (75%) would like to meet the donor[20]. It is not clear how the 36 respondents to the survey were recruited, but it might be assumed that they came from support groups and might, therefore, be more likely to oppose anonymity. Despite this probable bias, one-quarter of respondents were either unsure or did not want to know or meet the donor.

A number of press reports suggest that donor offspring, particularly adults, are keen to trace the donor and are extremely frustrated when they are unable to do so. But it could be argued that such views are more likely to be reported in the press because they contradict the status quo, and because adults at ease with their donor origin are less likely to feel the need to talk to the press. If they are happy not knowing the identity of their donor, they would probably feel no need to share this fact with the media.

We have very little information about what the offspring of anonymous donation, whether children or adults, feel about the fact that they will never meet the donor. We know that some are angry and upset about this, but we must also assume that there are as many – possibly more – who feel no such unhappiness or frustration. But if we have scant information about attitudes within anonymous donation, we have even less about attitudes within known donation. The assumption is sometimes made that everything is rosy in known donation: that donors, parents and offspring are happy and contented. But without more information, we cannot make this assumption and we cannot assess what impact known donation, perhaps involving a friend or a family member, has upon the child. More follow-up studies of people born of gamete donation (known and anonymous) are clearly needed before we can make an accurate diagnosis of the impact of the different systems on the welfare of the offspring. Without this information, we must assume that no significant harm is being done in either system.

A 'DOUBLE-TRACK' SYSTEM?

Pennings and others have argued for a 'double track' approach to the provision of donor conception services[8]. This means that both known and anonymous donation are available, both to donors and to the recipient prospective parents. While Pennings recognizes drawbacks in both systems, he suggests that the system

> 'represents the best attempt to balance the rights of donors, recipients and donor offspring. It offers the social parents the freedom to choose the degree to which they want the donor involved in their new family. It also enables donors to define their commitment'[8].

Is this an arrangement that prospective parents want? In the Netherlands, where a double track policy is currently in operation (though the anonymous strand is due to be phased out), the proportion of choices for either one or the other is about 50:50. In a recent study of Belgian egg donati recipients, 69% of couples opted for known donation, while 31% preferre anonymous donation[21]. These recipients were asked to recruit their ow donors and then offered a choice between using the eggs from their donor or using the eggs of an anonymous donor recruited by someone else. The authors note that the preference for known donation might reflect a willingness on the part of the donor to undergo an invasive procedure to help a couple they know, but an unwillingness to help a couple they do not know.

In a Dutch study of 38 families who had had children as a result of anonymous donor insemination, participants were asked whether, given the opportunity, they would have chosen anonymous donation with no information about the donor, donation with non-identifying information or known donation[22]. Of the 38 families 57% preferred anonymous donation; 31% would have opted for non-identifying information about the donor and 9% would have liked known donation (3% were unsure). The preference of these families for anonymous donation could be explained by the fact that they had already successfully conceived through this method.

These studies demonstrate that there certainly is variation in prospective parents' preference for known or anonymous donation. If we were to accept that it is the prospective parents who should decide upon the system of donation, it seems that the double track policy, offering a choice between known or anonymous donation, presents the best way of reflecting the variety of systems from which they would like to choose. What would happen if we had a system whereby all gametes were given by donors who were willing to be identified? This might be a system that would best please the offspring, because they could decide whether or not they wanted to trace the donor in the same way that adopted children can. The parents might not be satisfied, since they might have preferred an anonymous donor and no opportunity for tracing. But should the decision be the child's?

RESPECTING PROCREATIVE AUTONOMY

Pennings recognizes a number of limitations to his double track policy. One of these is that the 'system offers no solution to the problem of the children who wish to know the identity of their genetic parents'[8]. Wincott and Hedgley make a rather more obvious observation: 'Adults, whether infertile couples or potential donors, have choices ... But people born through assisted conception have no choice. They do not ask to be born'[5].

This, of course, is true of everybody. No one asked to be born: to do so would be impossible. As one newspaper comment put it: 'The fact is that parents are able to assume all kinds of things about the future wishes of the children for whom they take the responsibility of raising, from giving them unfortunate names to sending them to the wrong school'[23]. The rather trivial examples used here mask a more serious point. Adults make decisions on behalf of their future children all of the time: when they are born, who their parents are, how many siblings they have and, even, whether or not they are born. They also decide who the genetic parents are and whether the child will have contact with them. Harris argues that this is exactly what adults in a democratic society ought to be able to do[24]. Borrowing Dworkin's concept of procreative autonomy as based upon a belief in individual human dignity, Harris applies it to reproductive technologies:

> 'In so far as decisions to reproduce in particular ways or even using particular technologies constitute decisions concerning central issues of value, then arguably the freedom to make them is guaranteed ... by the constitution (written or not) of any democratic society, unless the state has a compelling reason for denying that control'[24].

Some might prefer an entirely known donation system in which the offspring of gamete donation decide whether or not to trace the donor. But this would mean that policy makers (by setting up the system) and offspring (in choosing to trace or not to trace) make decisions that ought to be the preserve of parents. This is tantamount to state denial of procreative autonomy; and because there is no evidence of harm to children born under known or anonymous donation, there can be no compelling reason for such an infringement of individual choice. One of Pennings's preferences for a double track policy is that 'it also expresses the idea that there is no unique and universal optimal solution'[8]. But we can go further than this. Both known and anonymous gamete donation are legitimate methods of having children, because neither does apparent harm to the offspring. But ultimately the optimal way of doing things is to leave the choice to the prospective parents. Apart from extreme circumstances (abuse, neglect etc.), child welfare is best promoted by allowing parents to make choices about their children.

If parents want the option of anonymous donation (which, from the studies discussed above, it seems they do), society should have a compelling reason to deny them that option. This principle applies equally to known donation: society should have a compelling reason to deny prospective parents that choice, too.

REFERENCES

1. Haimes E, Daniels K. International social science perspectives on donor insemination: an introduction. In: Daniels K, Haimes E, eds. *Donor Insemination: International Social Science Perspectives*. Cambridge: Cambridge University Press, 1998:1–6

2. Feversham report: report of the departmental committee on human artificial insemination. London: Her Majesty's Stationery Office, 1960: Cmnd 1105

3. Golombok S, Brewaeys A, Giavazzi MT, *et al*. The European study of assisted reproduction families: the transition to adolescence. *Hum Reprod* 2002: in press

4. Golombok S. *Parenting: What Really Counts?* London: Routledge, 2000:30–4

5. Wincott E, Hedgley T. Should sperm donors be traceable? *The Guardian*, 11 September 1999

6. Blyth E. Access to genetic origins information in donor-assisted conception: international perspectives. In: Blyth E, Crawshaw M, Speirs J, eds. *Truth and the Child 10 Years On: Information Exchange in Donor Assisted Conception*. Birmingham: British Association of Social Workers, 1998:69–78

7. Human Fertilisation and Embryology Authority. *Code of Practice*. London: HFEA, 2001

8. Pennings G. The 'double track' policy for donor anonymity. *Hum Reprod* 1997;12:2839–44

9. Congenital Disabilities (Civil Liability) Act 1976, s1A(1)

10. European Convention on Human Rights, articles 7 and 8

11. *R v Secretary of State for the Home Department ex parte Mellor*

12. McWhinnie A. Gamete donation and anonymity. *Hum Reprod* 2001;5:807–17

13. Smith J. Sperm donors have duties to their kids, too. *The Independent on Sunday*, 31 December 2000

14. Gottlieb C, Lalos O, Linkblad, F. Disclosure of donor insemination to the child: the impact of Swedish legislation on couples' attitudes. *Hum Reprod* 2000;9:2052–6

15. Jackson E. *Regulating Reproduction: Law, Technology and Autonomy*. Oxford: Hart Publishing, 2001

16. Dyer C. Offspring from artificial insemination demand fathers' details. *Br Med J* 2000;321:654

17. Tizzard J. New reproductive technologies: new ethical dilemmas and old moral prejudices. In: Lee E, ed. *The New Politics of Abortion*. London: Macmillan, 1998:184–97

18. Harris J. *The Value of Life*. London: Routledge, 1985:154

19. Turner AJ, Coyle A. What does it mean to be a donor offspring? *Hum Reprod* 2000;9:2041–51

20. Cordray B. Survey of people conceived through donor insemination. *Don Insem Network News* Winter 1999/2000

21. Baetens P, Devroey P, Camus M, *et al*. Counselling couples and donors for oocyte donation: the decision to use either known or anonymous oocytes. *Hum Reprod* 2000;2:476–84

22. Brewaeys A, Golombok S, Naaktgeboren N, *et al*. Donor insemination: Dutch parents' opinions about confidentiality and donor anonymity and the emotional adjustment of their children. *Hum Reprod* 1997;7:1591–7

23. Sperm donors should retain their right to anonymity. *The Independent*, 24 April 2000

24. Harris J. Rights and reproductive choice. In: Harris J, Holm S eds. *The Future of Human Reproduction: Ethics, Choice and Regulation*. Oxford: Clarendon Press, 1998:34–5

7

Cloning: reproductive, therapeutic or not at all?

F. Shenfield

INTRODUCTION

The argument in this chapter revolves around what is probably one of the most well known scientific techniques of the last decade – that of cloning. Public imagination was first captured in 1997 by the method of somatic cell nuclear transfer (SCNT) which led to the birth of Dolly, described by Wilmut and colleagues[1]. Since then fantastic interpretations of reproductive cloning in the human, and therapeutic hopes triggered by stem cell research, both in animals and in the human, have ensured continuous exposure of the term cloning worldwide. It seems that this terminology evokes as many concerns as hopes in the public at large, and particularly from the ethical point of view. This applies especially to reproductive cloning[2], but also has implications in the case of stem cells of any embryonic origin, even when this embryo does not originate from the SCNT technique. Politicians have been involved in the debates; national and international ethics committees have made pronouncements on the matter; bans have been called for; and hopes expressed of miraculous cures for diseases, all of which far outweigh the importance for health budgets of our specialty, namely the treatment of infertility. The whole subject of the ethical implications of stem cell techniques indeed deserves analysis, and several reports have been published already both nationally in the UK[3–5], France[6], Denmark[7] and Germany[8], as well as internationally[9].

However, the somewhat provocative title of this chapter refers to two specific aspects: human reproductive cloning, which has in practice been decried almost internationally, and stem cell techniques, whose hoped-for therapeutic applications have been hailed with a lot of excitement. These do not, at least now and in the foreseeable future, involve SCNT techniques in the majority of cases. At this stage SCNT represents only a theoretical variation on the embryonic stem cell technology in order to avoid the recipient's rejection occurring with the use of an allogenic source. Thus, for now the answer to the question in the title may well be: cloning? not at all, at least in the case of reproductive cloning, and certainly not yet for therapeutic cloning. Indeed the question itself is a plea for using proper terminology, not labeling all embryonic stem cell research as therapeutic cloning – especially when one is educating non-specialists who are then involved in decision making at regulatory level. It is hoped that a cogent argument for this proper semantic use follows in the two parts of this chapter, respectively about reproductive cloning and stem cell technology.

REPRODUCTIVE CLONING

In the case of the ethical analysis of reproductive cloning, there has been a renewed debate about the meaning of human identity for society, made even more topical at the time of writing as a team ready to flout all legal barriers and the concerns of many scientists about the safety of the technique itself has publicly announced its intention to attempt SCNT for human reproduction as soon as possible[10]. It is therefore still appropriate to analyze several responses triggered by the initial Dolly event, whether from philosophers, practitioners, scientists at the personal level, their representative societies at the professional level, or the larger societal frame as represented by national or international institutions.

The status of the human embryo (a potential for life, life itself?) has given rise to many debates, all of which have been rekindled by this recent scientific achievement. All different types of cloning, namely nuclear transplantation, blastomere separation, or bisection, elicit discomfort and raise the dangers of deliberate twinning. The term deliberate is crucial, as a deliberate action implies taking responsibility for that action. Hans Jonas based his ethical analysis on 'the responsibility principle', and stated that the responsibility of parents to their children is one of the most onerous we may face. This arguably may be extended to future or planned children, the matter which concerns us daily in assisted reproduction, and is probably the most important concern we have to keep in mind when contemplating reproductive cloning as well.

Nevertheless, most analysis published since 1997 rejected reproductive cloning on several different grounds. One may first instantly dismiss the often-used rationalizing 'nature' counter argument about the natural occurrence of identical twins ('Why do we object to cloning humans, as we do not object to the natural existence of spontaneous identical twins?'). Humans differ from other animals by their organization and integration into a social system, and scientists, doctors and carers of many qualifications commit themselves to a lifelong confrontation with the 'natural' events of illness and suffering, thus constantly reversing and tampering with nature.

Indeed, the report by the group of advisers to the European Union (GAEIB)[9] puts this notion in the following words: 'as there is no discrimination against twins *per se* it follows that there are no *per se* objections to genetically identical human beings'. It is to the planned creation of copies of individuals that objections have been raised, thus raising the question of a deliberate action, which implies our responsibility again.

What would be the objections to this deliberate planning? Threats to the notions of identity, dignity and uniqueness have been invoked in several reports in order to condemn human reproductive cloning, and must be further analyzed in order to assess the validity of all the objections offered.

The UNESCO declaration[11] on the genome places firmly the dignity of man within the context of uniqueness. The same argument of dignity is underlined by the French National Ethics Committee[12], which mainly concentrates on the identity problem. After stressing the absurdity entailed in considering 'the reductive illusion which is borne by the dismal confusion between identity in the physical sense of sameness and in the moral sense of self', it asserts however that reproductive cloning would still inaugurate a fundamental upheaval of the relationship between genetic identity and personal identity in its biological and cultural dimensions: 'creating (cloned) human beings, individuals in terms of their psyche in spite of their genetic similitude, would be seen in both the literal and the figurative senses of the word, as identical copies of each other and of the cloned individual of which they would truly be a copy'. Thus the threat to autonomy comes from the sense that the other person, or society as made by many different others, knowing they are clones would treat them as somewhat predetermined. This would entail a lack of liberty, even if relative but too awesome to contemplate for the future cloned person induced by this increase in genetic determinism.

One should also consider the psychological arguments: the narcissistic venture of the parent(s) threatens the building of the identity of the child, probably mostly by decreasing the possibility of separation from the initial model and his/her autonomy. While one is aware of the epigenetic differences with the model, it seems fair to be wary of the experiment from the point of view of identity in the broad sense, as well as the sexual sense. In the US report commissioned by President Clinton[13], 'fears about harms to the children who may be created in this manner, particularly psychological harms associated with a possibly diminished sense of individuality and personal autonomy' belong to the same analysis.

One must also add consideration of the social dimension of the individual, as the integration to a social system characterizes the human as a species. We need therefore to analyze the other two main objections in the realms of societal interaction, made by several reports: respectively the danger of instrumentalization, either by one person or a group, of another person and the danger of eugenics.

We have seen that the notions of autonomy and respect are used as tools to object to reproductive cloning, but treating the person as an object is a concern present in both the US report and the European report from the EU experts. Eugenics may arguably be considered as an extreme form of instrumentalization, not between one person and another, but between one group of persons and another group, considered inferior in their differences. Amongst the 'potential harm to important social values', the National Bioethics Advisory Commission (NBAC) report qualifies eugenics as 'a path that humanity has tread before, to its everlasting shame'. However, the American Engelhardt[14] is a dissenting voice with a very liberal discourse. He argues that positive eugenics is totally within the principles of autonomy and beneficence when he states 'if there is nothing sacred about human nature, there is no reason why, with proper reasons and proper caution, it should not be radically changed'.

All in all, in the face of this international rejection of reproductive cloning, national instruments have therefore been used. National instruments are often legal, a much stronger statement than just a code of practice for professionals. Some countries have opted to define and ban cloning in their national laws by reference to a given technique (embryo splitting or nuclear transfer), others have avoided this difficulty by banning cloning whatever process is used. International instruments, however, are necessarily general in scope and often purely declamatory[15]. Such an instance is the added protocol to the Council of Europe Convention for the Protection of Human Rights and Dignity of the Human Being with regard to the application of Biology and Medicine[16] (Convention on Human Rights and Biomedicine), on the prohibition of cloning human beings. This was signed on 12th January 1998, in Paris, by several members of the Council of Europe.

Finally, both the US and European reports stress the importance of educating the public in order to enable a more democratic process of decision making. The European Commission is indeed 'invited to stimulate the debate involving public, consumers, patients, environment and animal protection associations, and a well structured public debate should be set up at European level'. As for the Council of Europe Bioethics Convention, it expresses the need for international co-operation 'so that all humanity may enjoy the benefits of biology and medicine'. A major problem has arisen from the terminology used about therapeutic cloning in general.

In France, for instance, the belated revision of the 1994 legislation which is expected to be presented soon to the parliamentary chambers is still restricted in its approach to embryo research[17]. Many arguments in the debate leading to the proposal for law reform seem to be linked to the much exposed 'slippery slope' argument centering on the word cloning. This argument seems to imply that if therapeutic cloning were to be allowed, it would inevitably lead to condoning reproductive cloning. The concerns about embryo cloning for reproduction in general and the identical name used in discussions in reproductive cloning and the SCNT technique described as cloning induce the fear that the former will follow the latter without fail.

Arguing from the standpoint of dangers of reproductive cloning it becomes easy to demand a total ban on the use of embryos for stem cell research, as has been seen recently in the USA. It then becomes much more difficult to explain and publicize new stem cell technologies and their potential. Finally and most importantly, it becomes more difficult to analyze the different ethical problems, which indeed vary according to the source of the stem cells.

STEM CELL RESEARCH

In the case of the stem cell debate, the embryo is still at the core of the debate, because of its symbolic representation of our future. But the repulsion caused almost universally by reproductive cloning has not been universally matched by the same feelings or arguments on the use of stem cells from embryos. However, at this moment Britain may be the only country which allows therapeutic cloning[18], while the French do not envisage this possibility. The revised law plans to allow the use of spare embryos from ART cycles for research on pluripotent cells. But it does not involve allowing research on the spare embryos in order to improve ART itself. The irony is that this approach is both more utilitarian than principled and penalizes infertile patients. This is surprising indeed in a country where moral principles are not unusually used in legal parlance, as for instance in the introduction to the 1994 laws which mentions 'respect' (owed to human life). And also because France is an example of good egalitarian access to treatment for the infertile, certainly compared to the UK where only two couples out of ten have free National Health Service access to *in vitro* fertilization, despite the government's undertaking to change[19].

In the UK embryo research has been licensed under strict conditions since the HFE Act 1990[20], permitting only research linked to reproduction. After a democratic process involving a report by the Chief Medical Officer[4] and a vote in both parliamentary chambers, new categories were added to Statute Jan 31st 2001, allowing 'research for serious disease'. Interestingly, in a bid to slow the licensing of this new application, a 'pro-life' lobby has asked a judge[21] to assess whether an embryo created by SCNT would actually qualify to be such an entity in terms of the HFE Act 1990. Surprisingly, the High Court actually ruled on November 15th 2001 that this entity is not an embryo under the Act (it would be another kind of embryo, and if so which kind?). The logical consequence would be that the protection or framework offered by the amended statute does not then apply, and the argument that the danger of reproductive cloning still looms large would prevail, or at least be used by the pro-life alliance. The situation would then be similar to what occurred when the term 'pre-embryo' was used. This term was heavily criticized, especially in Europe, in words that can be summarized by the laconic label of a philosopher member of the French National Ethics Committee decrying the terminology as circumstantial ontology[22]. This may be followed later by other attempts at semantic games in order to use the embryo in research of yet another kind, and does not bode well for either scientific integrity or transparency. Whatever our leanings, whether more deontological or utilitarian, most agents involved in the debate would probably agree that honesty and truthfulness are virtues not to be sacrificed. It seems therefore honest to say that an embryo is an embryo however it was created, even if not replaced in the uterus. However, the British Government's response was to publish a one-line Bill barring reproductive cloning, which has already been passed in both Houses and awaits Royal assent. Finally, allowing the Government's appeal to the 'pro-life' case[21], the Court of Appeal ruled that a cloned embryo does fall within the legal definition of an embryo, despite the fact that fertilization has not technically taken place. The judges argued that the spirit of the law was intended to include cloned embryos. Lord Phillips added that 'if parliament had known of the cloning technique in 1990 it would certainly have been included in the legislation which controls research and use of embryos'[23]. Another approach is that of the Infertility Treatment Authority in the state of Victoria[24], which stated that 'ES cells ... are not the equivalent of an intact embryo ... as a clump of ES cells transferred to a uterus would not become a viable fetus'. As the Victoria Act[25] forbids destructive research on embryos, it means that in this case the definition of an embryo according to the Act does not apply to ES cells, and research on them is therefore not illegal in Victoria. But this is different to stating that the embryo, before its blastocyst stage and potential stem cells, does not deserve its name if created in a certain way, as for example by SCNT.

Aware of the potential exploitation of these semantic games, the European Society for Human Reproduction and Embryology (ESHRE) task force[26] defined the preimplantation embryo in its first ethics consideration on behalf of the society. The task force stressed that this term was descriptive, referring to the embryo out of the body before it is given a chance of becoming a fetus and then a legal person by ET. But such a descriptive term does not imply a lesser quality. We practitioners and scientists should not use semantic particularities which will allow opponents to any kind of research to deride professionals who might simply rename the entity embryo in order to make the consequences of its use more acceptable. The difficulties outlined here are illustrated by the many different national legal definitions[27] of the embryo for statutory purposes, whilst there is usually no definition of the beginning of life. At international level declarations often use symbolic language, which complicates matters even further, as it is extremely difficult to reconcile the pragmatic and the symbolic.

Meanwhile, we must be pragmatic if we are to analyze the ethical issues arising from the possible application of stem cell animal research to the human embryo, and assume at least that we can consider this source acceptable in order to assess the dangers as well as the exciting possibilities. With this in mind the ESHRE task force on law and ethics recently considered the matter of stem cell technology[28]. Essential to the analysis is the definition of a stem cell as "a cell which retains the ability to self renew and to differentiate into one or several cell types". Stem cells may be derived from the embryo, the fetus or the adult, but our purpose, in this chapter dedicated to cloning, is to concentrate on the ethical issues from embryonic stem (ES) cells derived from the blastocyst. Thus the task force also endeavors to distinguish the research on and possible use of several types of embryonic stem cells: those issued from blastocysts either supernumerary or created *de novo* and those created by nuclear transfer from somatic cells. The latter method is usually referred to as cloning, although this refers here to the method resulting in the birth of the sheep Dolly, where only the nucleus of the daughter cell is identical to that of the original somatic cell while the cytoplasm is that of the recipient enucleated oocyte. We see that this is different to the definition of cloning which implies regeneration of totally identical cells starting from one cell only. Indeed this method should be called SCNT. The first point to be made is that there is a lack of knowledge about safety, itself a major ethical problem. But notwithstanding the current technical problems, and especially for now the scarcity of human studies, the lack of data on factors controlling specific differentiation; the theoretical danger of neoplasia or tumor formation; and in the case of somatic cell nuclear transfer, the questions about the normality of ES cells from cloned blastocysts, the task force endeavors to analyze the other ethical issues involved in ES cell technology, whatever their source. These issues are summarized below.

Some fundamental ethical questions in this field are far from new. Indeed consent must be obtained for research, reflecting the principle of autonomy. However, the task force stresses 'in view of the special nature of stem cells and their longevity, it should be specifically mentioned that the embryos will be used for research into the establishment of cell lines which can be kept indefinitely, may eventually be used for therapeutic purposes, and will never be replaced into a uterus. It should also be made clear whether the cells may be used for commercial and/or clinical purposes'. This is therefore specific rather than general consent.

There are also specific ethical considerations according to the source of the cells, and especially regarding the creation of embryos specifically for research. The ESHRE ethics task force first considerations on ethics and law on the preimplantation embryo states 'we do not object to embryo research on supernumerary embryos nor do we find any major ethical differences with embryos created for research within (specific) constraints. The constraint imposed is essential however: the creation and the possibility of research on preimplantation embryos specifically created for the purpose is appropriate only if the information cannot be obtained by research on supernumerary zygotes'[26]. As we know, this question of the creation of embryos for research is especially vexed. While article 18 of the European Convention on Human Rights and Biomedicine specifically forbids this, in the UK the HFEA is charged with overseeing embryo research within the limits by a licensing system. It is not forbidden in the UK to create embryos *de novo* for research, but with a similar caveat, ensuring that embryos are not created for futile reasons.

Other issues are also of grave concern. For instance, the question of patenting evokes a number of ethical and legal questions. The proposed declaration of the task force emphasizes that 'the patenting policy should not hamper the development of new technologies or slow down the acquisition of knowledge. Given the huge potential benefits for a considerable number of patients suffering from various diseases, the health of the population in general should take priority over commercial goals. Moreover, patenting should not unduly restrict the fundamental principle of freedom of research. However, in practice the specific issue of the source of the oocytes used for any embryos created for the purpose of research is a major problem in view of the already well documented imbalance between needs and supply in the case of egg donation.' As there is a limited number of oocytes available should they preferentially be allocated to reproduction? Potential abuse of vulnerable women who might be enticed to sell their oocytes for research is certainly a grave concern, as it has been for several years in the field of gametes donation.

At European level, though, the European Group on Ethics (EGE) has been more conservative in its recommendations, made public in November 2000[29]. It stresses again in its final report the latest addition to the European corpus, in the fundamental Charter of Rights of the European Union approved by the European Council of Biarritz in October 2000, which forbids reproductive cloning. But it deems ethically unacceptable the creation of embryos from donated gametes, because surpernumerary embryos are an alternative available source. In the case of embryos obtained by SCNT, it voices its extreme concern, while aware that 'the creation of (such) embryos may be the most effective way of obtaining pluripotent stem cells genetically identical to the patient's and thus obtaining perfectly compatible tissues with the aim of avoiding rejection after transplantation'. The prime objection concerns the danger of exploiting women donors: these remote therapeutic perspectives must be balanced with the risks of embryo trivialization, and of exerting pressure on women as sources of oocytes, and increasing the possibility of their instrumentalization. It finally considers that it applies the principle of proportionality by adopting a cautious approach, and itself qualifies its own approach by the word 'prudence', taking into account that there is already 'a vast field of research to explore with the other sources of stem cells'.

The EGE also recommends that EU funding should be made available, within the usual framework of research, and also specifically tackles the concerns of research in this field. Specifically it mentions 'the free and informed consent of donors and of recipients, and for the possible use of the embryo cells for the specific purpose in question'; and 'the need to protect the anonymity of donors while retaining the ability of donors and recipients to be traced in case unsatisfactory side-effects occur'.

CONCLUSIONS

Thus we may conclude that many consider stem cells from embryos created by SCNT a feminist issue because the main danger lies in the exploitation of women, enticing them to relinquish oocytes by coercion. This is a fair comment at a time when the disproportion between donation of and demand for oocytes is prevalent everywhere, although this objection may be rethought if/when IVM becomes a better source of oocytes. The compromise wait and see attitude of the EGE may be seen as wise, or as lacking in vision, but it certainly addresses all the issues in depth. Nevertheless scientists in the field agree that research should continue with all sources of stem cells, as we cannot yet know which source – if any – is going to fulfill the therapeutic promise. We note the recent compromise agreed by the Bush administration to allow public funds to be used for research only on existing cells lines[30]. While an understandable political compromise on the US scene, it is remote from the sense of responsibility generally expressed in Europe, whether towards the fate of supernumerary embryos, or the more contentious subject of the creation of embryos for the purpose of research. But most importantly attempts to discredit embryo research in general should be resisted, as there already exist several models of licensing statutory framework which function with enough safeguards to reassure society at large.

REFERENCES

1. Wilmut I, Schnieke AE, McWhir J, *et al*. Viable offspring derived from fetal and adult mammary cells. *Nature* 1987;387:810–13
2. Shenfield F, ed. Cloning: societal, medical and ethical implications of cloning. Presented at a workshop held at the Royal Society, London, 12 Jan 1999. European Commission, Science, Research and Development, Eur 18 180
3. *Stem cell therapy: the ethical issues, a discussion paper*. Nuffield Council on Bioethics, London, 2000

4.   *Stem cell research: medical progress with responsibility*. London: Department of Health. June 2000 (www.doh.gov.uk)
5.   *Stem cell research – second update*. The Royal Society, Policy document 9/01, June 2001, London
6.   Le clonage, la thérapie cellulaire et l'utilisation thérapeutique des cellules embryonnaires. Office parlementaire d'évaluation des choix scientifiques et technologiques, no 2198, Assemblée Nationale, no 238 Senat
7.   Skovmand K. Danish council votes yes to research into therapeutic cloning. *Lancet* 2001;357:780
8.   Abbott A. Stem cell research delayed by German ethics council. *Nature* 2001; 411:875
9.   McLaren A. European Union European Commission, 28 May 1997. Opinion of the group of advisors on the Ethical Implications of Biotechnology to the European Commission: Ethical Aspects of Cloning Techniques
10. Vogel G. Human cloning plans spark talk of US ban. *Science* 2001;292:31
11. *Universal declaration on the human genome*, UNESCO, 11 Nov 1997, 11, Place de Fontenoy, Paris
12. CCNE, Réponse au Président de la République au sujet du clonage reproductif, cahiers du CCNE, Paris, 1997
13. National Bioethics Advisory Commission report to the President of the United States of America, June 9th 1997
14. Hottois, G. In: Jones H, Engelhardt HT, eds. *Aux Fondements d'une Ethique Contemporaine*. Paris: Librairie Philosophique Jean Vrin, 1993:143–56
15. Le Bris S, Hirtle M. Report prepared for GAIEB. Les aspects éthiques et juridiques du clonage humain: perspectives comparatives. Centre de Recherche en Droit Public, Faculté de Droit, Montréal, 1997
16. Added protocol to the Convention for the Protection of Human Rights and Dignity of the Human Being with Regard to the Application of Biology and Medicine. Paris: 13 January, 1998
17. Nau JY. Le parlement s'apprête à autoriser les recherches sur l'embryon. *Le Monde*, 15 January, 2002
18. *The Human Reproductive Cloning Act*, 2001, London: HMSO, 2001: www.legislation.hmso.gov.uk
19. Shenfield F. Justice and access to fertility treatments. In: Shenfield F, Sureau C, eds. *Ethical Dilemmas in Assisted Reproduction*. Carnforth, UK: Parthenon Publishing, 1997:4–16
20. *Human Fertilisation and Embryology Act 1990*. London: HMSO, 1990
21. The Queen on the application of Pro Life Alliance v. Secretary of State for Health CO/4095/2000
22. Seve L. Pour une critique de la raison bioéthique. Paris: Editions Odile Jacob, 1994
23. *The Independent*, 19 January, 2002
24. Infertility Treatment Authority, 2000. The use of embryonic stem cells. www.ita.org.au
25. Infertility Treatment Act 1995
26. ESHRE taskforce on law and ethics. I. The moral status of the pre-implantation embryo. *Hum Reprod* 16;1046–8
27. IFFS Surveillance 98. *Fertil Steril* 1999;71(S)

28. ESHRE SIG Ethics and Law. Ethical considerations: Stem cells (14 May 2001) www.eshre.com
29. The European Group on Ethics in Science and New Technologies to the European Commission (2000). Adoption of an opinion on ethical aspects of human cell research and use, Paris, 14 Nov 2000, revised edition Jan 2001, Secretariat of the Group, Brussels
30. Bonetta L. Storm in a culture dish. *Nature* 2001;413:345–6

8

The fetus as a patient: wrongful life, wrongful death

C. Sureau and F. Shenfield

INTRODUCTION

For many years now obstetricians have considered the fetus as a prenatal 'patient'. In fact this recognition goes back to the 19th century (1821) when J.A. Lejumeau de Kergaradec, trying to hear the noise produced by the amniotic fluid, through a Laennec stethoscope, was surprised to get a 'double' beat. He was able to deduce its fetal cardiac origin and genius enough to speculate that the fetus' state of health or illness could be evaluated according to the strength and rhythm of the heart beat. This discovery led to a fundamental change: the fetus was no more a kind of thing, sometimes an obstacle, which had to be removed in order to rescue the mother, but a living being, which (or who) may need help and assistance[1].

Years later fetal medicine began when fetal–maternal biological conflict due to Rhesus incompatibility was understood, explained, treated and finally prevented, and when medical treatments of fetal diseases were initiated, or surgical interventions undertaken. This evolution shows clearly that since the early beginning of gestation the 'child to be' is considered by the obstetrician/perinatologist as a patient, from a medical standpoint.

However, this medical attitude is by no means linked to philosophical or legal judgments about fetal personhood.

Chervenak and McCullough have offered several very interesting reflections about the philosophical and ethical aspects of the question[2]. For them, the fetus is to be considered as a patient when it becomes viable, and it is only at that time that its interests and rights ought to be taken into consideration. Before the time of viability the potential survival of the fetus (and earlier of the embryo) depends solely on the maternal decision. As Chervenak and McCullough say 'the previable fetus is presented to the physician solely as a function of the pregnant woman's autonomy'. Conversely, after the deadline of viability 'a pregnant woman is obliged to take only reasonable risks with obstetric interventions that are reliably expected to benefit the viable fetus or child later'[2].

This is not the place to discuss this opinion, which reflects the classical reference to the concept of autonomy, sometimes in opposition to the one of beneficence. Suffice it to say how weak and imprecise is this threshold of viability, which depends on so many factors, and is more a statistical concept than a factual one in medical situations[3]. This is particularly so when considering not only the medical or the ethical but also the legal aspects. When trying to consider the viability of a fetus from a legal standpoint, it is frequently (in the 'borderline' situations) difficult to determine if viability was possible (some fetuses of 19 weeks or 320 g have survived), probable (value over a 50% threshold?), or certain. The consequences of survival may also be considered, as indeed may the threshold of survival without disability, which may also modify medical decisions.

Consequently the matter appears to be particularly complex and several questions arise. Is it pertinent to use the concept of a threshold of supposed viability to state precisely the kind of responsibility engaged in the loss of a viable fetus *in utero*? Moreover might such a negligent loss entail the crime of homicide? Conversely what are the civil rights of an embryo or fetus? Is it possible to consider either as a person, entailing what the French call subjective rights (*'des droits subjectifs'*)? Do these rights include the right to live (or die), according to the decision of the mother, and up to what term of pregnancy, keeping in mind that such rights could lead to penal prosecution or civil liability if not respected?

These questions have been debated at length in the past in several countries. Several court decisions have recently been issued in France, which may lead to meaningful reflections, since they occurred in a country which bears two characteristics. One derives from the legal standpoint, the reference to statute law which, as in numerous countries of continental Europe, is influenced by the Roman legal system in opposition to natural law. The second characteristic is from the ethical standpoint: preference is frequently given to the concept of beneficence over the principle of autonomy. Interestingly enough it will be shown that despite these apparent differences a convergent evolution between statute and common law may be observed.

WRONGFUL DEATH

The question arises: may an accidental fetal death *in utero* be considered as a homicide, namely a criminal offence, from the legal standpoint? Several answers have been given to this fundamental question. In Germany such a prosecution concerning a fetus cannot be accepted (decision of the Federal Constitutional Court, July 29, 1988). Prosecution can only ensue when a newborn is concerned, or if a fetus dies during the course of delivery (#222. Penal Code).

brief /examination

In Spain there is also no prosecution for homicide in case of fetal death, but specific prosecution for injuries to a fetus (Art. 157. Penal Code) or abortion caused by imprudence (Art. 146. Penal Code) may be started. On May 10th 1999, this article 146 was invoked in a case of abortion carried out owing to violence against the mother.

In Italy homicide may be considered only when fetal death occurred between the separation of the fetus from the uterus and birth. Abortion provoked accidentally does not fit within this definition, but is submitted to a special penalty (Art. 17, law 22.5.78). In the Netherlands there is no prosecution in such a situation. In the United Kingdom, as in most of the countries of common law, the legal personhood of the fetus is not recognized. Consequently the suit of manslaughter cannot be applied.

In the USA specific prosecution may be initiated for injury to the fetus in 24 different states, with or without reference to the term of pregnancy. Some states refer to the old-fashioned term of 'quickening', 18 of them, in agreement with the common law (born alive rule), do not give any special protection to the fetus and six states limit their penal intervention to the case of specific violence against the mother.

In France two court decisions have been issued, which will be briefly mentioned. On June 30th 1999 a decision of the Criminal Chamber of the Cassation Court (i.e. the supreme court for civil or criminal affairs) involved a case of confusion between two Vietnamese patients with the same name, neither of whom spoke French, one attending for the removal of an intrauterine contraceptive device (IUCD), the other for amniocentesis at 21–22 weeks. The attempted removal of the IUCD in the pregnant patient provoked the rupture of membranes, followed by the intrauterine death of the fetus and the need for evacuation. At first instance the suit for homicide was denied by the court, but the Court of Appeal accepted the concept of homicide. In the final instance, the Cassation Court revoked this 'because Article 221.6 of the Penal Code defines precisely homicide in French law (i.e. the fact to cause the death of '*autrui*', i.e. somebody else) and that the fetus is not this somebody else'. A fundamental principle of French law is that the interpretation of the Penal Code is strict, that it cannot be submitted to extrapolation, interpretation or assimilation (principle of 'legality'). However, doubt remained owing to the fact that this particular fetus was not considered viable, and that in another case where a car crash resulted in the death of an 8-months fetus the Court of Appeal (Reims, 3.2.2000) had accepted the qualification of homicide (but with no further referral to the Cassation Court).

On June 29th 1995 another car crash caused the death of a 6-months fetus *in utero*. The Court of Appeal (Metz, 3.09.1998) refused the qualification of homicide, and the case was brought to the Cassation Court, which gave its sentence in plenary formation (a special disposition reinforcing the strength of the judiciary decision, which then becomes a principle of law). The decision of the court was that, again, the Penal Code must be interpreted strictly, literally and not with approximation and that the word homicide written in the Penal Code (Art. 221.6) cannot refer to the fetus *in utero*. This decision was taken without reference to fetal viability at the time of death. Thus, this important judgment appears to be in agreement with most court decisions in different national jurisdictions, and involves three concepts:

(1) One of a medical nature, the concept of viability, useful in medical practice, but established on statistical retrospective studies.

(2) One of legal nature: the limitation of acknowledgement of personhood to the 'born alive', in agreement with the legal system of most countries of common law, at least from the penal point of view. From the civil point of view the situation may be slightly different since, according to the Roman rule *'infans conceptus pro nato habetur quoties de commodo ejus'*, the beginning of personhood and civil rights may be retrospectively established back to the time of conception, provided it is born living and viable, and if it is in its own interest.

(3) Finally one of ethical nature, which leads to a position rather different from the one expressed by Chervenak and McCullough, since it does not refer to the concept of viability.

This is of the utmost importance ethically: although there are differences between common and statutory law, with a tighter link between ethics and law in the former than in the latter, the same problem persists, which is the definition of the beginning of human life and of ethical, or possibly legal, personhood.

Some will consider, mainly for philosophical reasons or religious beliefs, that conception is the key point; it follows that any destruction of embryonic or fetal life is a homicide at any time, or even in any anatomical situation. This attitude will, of course, include early voluntary abortion, whether instrumental or medical, but also the use of IUCDs, even embryo destruction in case of ectopic pregnancy, and obviously destruction of cryopreserved embryos or research on embryos or embryonic cells. Beside this extreme position exists a wide range of attitudes, from the acceptance of all or only some medical and scientific advances. One attitude is proposed by Chervenak and McCullough, who give absolute autonomy to the mother up to fetal viability, then impose on her shared responsibility for herself and for the fetus, with the possibility of ensuing conflicts.

It is interesting to note that in France a conceptual evolution is taking place. While legal and moral concepts are readily mixed, and protection of the future baby's life began at conception (Art. 1 of 1975 law on voluntary abortion, Art. 2 of the 1994 laws on *in vitro* fertilization and related matters, and Article 16 of the Civil Code) within the exclusively dualistic

Roman reference of persons and things, there has been recognition and the acceptance of a specific status (legal, and more precisely penal, for the time being) for the embryo and the fetus.

WRONGFUL LIFE

Three 'prejudices' may be associated with pregnancy and birth[4]. Wrongful conception may result from a preceding medical mistake, either wrong advice about the risk of transmission of a congenital disease (Cass. Civ. 26. 6.96), or the result of failure of sterilization or of interruption of pregnancy, but without any consequence on the physical state of the child (Conseil d'État, 2.07.82; Cass. Civ. 25.6.91). In France the general rule is to acknowledge that life *per se* cannot be considered as damage, nor lead to liability either from a penal or even a civil point of view. There are a few exceptions such as, for example, the impact of being born as a result of rape or incest with psychological injury (Cass. Crim. 4.2.98).

Damages may be awarded to the parents when the birth is linked to deleterious consequences of an obstetric accident, during either pregnancy or delivery. This prejudice is recognized everywhere, and leads to compensation. Markesinis pointed out its major problem: one must avoid double compensation for the same prejudice (i.e. it is legitimate to consider the psychologic trouble for the parents, as well as their special expenses to take care of the injured child, in addition to their normal obligation to him or her; but the addition of wrongful life prejudice would mean duplication of the damages). Another difficulty is the duration of the allocation of resources; should this be during the lifetime of the parents, up to the majority of the child, or for the whole life of the child?

The wrongful life concept is more subtle, the word itself being used more or less specifically in the US.

There is a relatively wide range of decisions concerning this type of prejudice. Although many wrongful birth actions have been accepted by different US courts (Custodio versus Bauer, California 1967; Shelton versus St Anthony's Medical Center, Missouri 1989; Breman versus Allen, New Jersey 1979), some have been rejected (Taylor versus Kurapati, Michigan 1999; courts in Idaho, Indiana, South Dakota, Minnesota, Pennsylvania; Georgia [Etkind versus Suarez, Georgia 1999], Ohio [Hester versus Dwivedi, Simmerer versus Dabbas, 1999]). However, most of the wrongful life actions have been rejected, resulting in eight states forbidding such actions by statute law. Only a few states have accepted the principle of compensation in such cases, but with very important restrictions: California (Gamy versus Mulliken. Med. Cent, 1993), only for 'economic damages', Washington and New Jersey (Procanik versus Cillo, 1984) for 'extraordinary medical or educational expenses'.

In the UK the same very restrictive attitude has been adopted. Compensation for injuries occurring before birth is dealt with under the Congenital Disability (civil liability) Act (1976) which excludes a suit against the mother. This was confirmed in the decision of the Court of Appeal of 1982 (McKay versus Essex Area Authority). The same principle applies in Belgium, the Netherlands, Israel, Quebec and Scandinavian countries. In Germany the Constitutional Court differentiated in 1997 between life *per se*, which cannot be considered as a prejudice, and the necessity of special care which must be compensated for the parents. In France compensation was given (27.9.89, Conseil d'État) to a child born with a missing limb because of medical fault arising from an unsuccessful abortion. This was generally considered fair, but since then several more recent cases have come to the attention of the public and the medical and legal professions, showing again an interesting merging between legal and ethical concepts.

They involve first the Quarez case, settled by the Conseil d'État, February 14, 1997. It is worth noting the specific jurisdictional situation prevailing in France: although all criminal prosecutions and civil affairs involving private persons are dealt with by the usual courts (1st instance Tribunal, Appeal and Cassation Court if necessary), cases concerning relationships involving private persons and state administration (including public hospitals which belong to the state or city administration) are dealt with by first degree administrative courts, then administrative Courts of Appeal and finally in appeal to the Conseil d'État. This double hierarchy of courts leads sometimes to 'conflicts of doctrine', as the following cases will show.

Mrs Quarez had been delivered of a trisomy 21 child after a failed diagnosis due to administrative error, with the consequence that she did not choose a termination of pregnancy (TOP), which she would have elected if correctly informed. The hospital was ordered to give damages to the parents, mainly for psychologic distress, and also to pay a special monthly allocation of resources to cover extra expenses incurred during the whole life of the child. With this decision the Conseil d'État took into consideration the special needs of the child, but refused to consider that the child was suffering from a prejudice of life, and specifically that no life would have been better than this life.

However, the Perruche case has recently challenged this thinking[5]. Mrs Perruche caught rubella from her daughter while pregnant, requested antenatal diagnosis and stated that she would request a TOP if infected. Laboratory and medical errors led to the birth of a severely affected baby boy. The legal situation was unusual since after a first instance trial, a first court of appeal considered that the doctor and laboratory were not liable, since they were not directly responsible for the rubella. The Court of Cassation (civil chamber) revoked the decision in 1996 and referred the case to another court of appeal, which then 'rebelled' by confirming the decision of the first court of appeal without taking the hint from the Cassation Court. In such a situation the case has to come back to the plenary assembly of the Court of Cassation, which confirmed on November 17 2000 the decision of the civil chamber. This decision was founded on the basis that without the medical mistake the pregnancy would have been terminated and that consequently the medical mistake was responsible for the prejudice. Following this reasoning the court awarded damages to the parents and damages directly to the child. This decision, particularly when compared to the decision of the Conseil d'État in the Quarez case, led to a considerable amount of discussion, not only from the legal and ethical points of view but also from the medical point of view.

From the legal point of view, the opposite attitudes of both courts arose owing to a differing consideration of the link of causation, a pragmatic link for the Cassation Court – i.e. without the mistake, the disability would have been avoided since an abortion would have occurred. A direct causative link was denied by the Conseil d'État since the damage was not due to medical error but to genetic abnormality.

From the moral point of view the decision of the Conseil d'État was considered hypocritical by some since it recognized the fetal need for compensation without saying it clearly; the decision of the court in the Perruche case was considered dangerous and questionable for the following reasons: recognition de facto of a right to die, or of a life of inferior value, in contradiction to human dignity, as firmly stated by several associations of parents of disabled children; and the danger of future trials against parents in the name of the child. Fear was expressed of a further increase in the number of court cases, particularly for ultrasound misdiagnosis of fetal abnormalities, and of an increased demand for medically indicated TOP because of doctors' and parents' fear of trials by children born damaged.

Furthermore, a more recent decision of the Court of Cassation (July 13, 2001)[6] which denied the liability of doctors who had missed the diagnosis of congenital abnormalities (spina bifida with hydrocephalus, missing segments of arms) was relatively reassuring in this respect. However, the court confirmed that, provided proof of a direct causal relationship is brought, a compensation is to be obtained by a child with a handicap for prejudice of life. The Cassation Court took into consideration the direct link of the fault with the lack of termination, instead of the direct link of the fault with the disability as requested by the Conseil d'État.

CONCLUSION

These recent cases are of paramount interest since they reflect a slow evolution of thought from both legal and ethical points of view[7–8]. It is more and more accepted that the principle of causation must be analyzed and applied in a very pragmatic way, depending on the specific situation, bearing in mind that the medical profession submits to an obligation of means and not of result. When a medical fault is demonstrated with deleterious consequences for the child, it is legitimate for the parents to obtain compensation; the child is also to be compensated for its suffering and for the care it will need during his/her whole life; however, this compensation is a function of the prejudice suffered and not the actual life.

It remains to be determined if disabled children in general – including those whose abnormality involves a medical liability – are to be better covered for their extra living expenses through the help of society at large, by democratic solidarity through structures included in national health service systems, or by medical liability and lawsuits. Europe in general favors the former approach.

As an example of this attitude, the French Parliament ruled in February 2002 that compensation for a congenital handicap can be obtained by the child only if the handicap is directly linked to medical negligence. However, in cases where failure to detect a handicap during pregnancy prevents the parents asking for a TOP, the parents may only obtain compensation for their own prejudice. Furthermore, this compensation cannot include the expenses covering the consequences of this handicap during the lifetime of their child, as these expenses have to be covered by a national solidarity system.

The final point, which correlates well with the notion of respect for the embryo stressed in the chapter concerning the obtaining of stem cells, is that here too there should appear an acknowledgment of a specific status for the embryo and fetus.

REFERENCES

1. Sureau C. Historical perspectives: forgotten past, unpredictable future. In: Gardosi J, ed. Intrapartum surveillance. *Baillière's Clin Obstet Gynaecol* 1996; 10:167–84
2. Chervenak FA, McCullough LB. Ethics in fetal medicine. In: Sureau C, Kohane-Shenfield F, eds. Ethical problems in obstetrics and gynaecology. *Baillière's Best Pract Res* 1999;13:491–502
3. Sureau C. Subsidiairement: réflexions sur la pertinence du concept de viabilité. *Responsabilité* 2001;3:30–3
4. Kennedy I, Grubb A. *Prenatal Injuries and Action for Wrongful Life and Wrongful Birth, Medical Law, Text and Materials.* London: Butterworth, 1998:817
5. Markesinis B. Réflexions d'un comparatiste anglais sur et à partir de l'arrêt Perruche. RTD civ, janv-mars, 2001:77–102
6. Sureau C. Le médecin et les naissances préjudiciables. In: Juger LV, Jaannet P, Iacub M, eds. *La Découverte* 2001:93–110
7. Steinbock B. The logical case for 'wrongful life'. *Hastings Center Report* 1986: 15–20
8. Steinbock B. When is birth unfair to the child? *Hastings Center Report* 1994: 15–21

9

Conclusion: cultural diversity, but common goals

F. Shenfield and C. Sureau

A major feature emerging from the different chapters of this book is a diversity of approach, which often reflects cultural diversity and different philosophical approaches or religious traditions. This diversity, striking even when considering medical attitudes to assisted human reproduction, both worldwide and within the continent of Europe, has sometimes been deplored. The fact that similar therapeutic approaches are not readily available in different parts of the world or Europe has been criticized, for two main reasons. The first reason is rather theoretical: it is argued that the continued existence of local characteristics in this field contributes to slow down the process of cohesion in the European Community. This argument is by no means convincing since, even in specific countries, different cultural behaviors may be observed in various regions. The second objection may appear more powerful: it concerns the risk of what has been labeled 'procreative tourism'. That some women (and/or couples) have to cross national borders in order to obtain a different assisted reproduction technology (ART) technique that they cannot obtain locally may be considered totally unethical.

An apparently similar situation occurred in the past when women sought voluntary abortions outside their legal national framework, something they still endeavor to do if they fall foul of the time limit for terminations where they reside. However, the degree of emergency, the social and economic considerations, the stress of necessity and the difficulties of travelling are of quite different magnitudes in the two situations. Moreover this diversity of approaches may and probably must be considered as a positively enriching feature, as indeed it is stated by both the European Union and the Council of Europe in several documents. Furthermore, diversity may be a factor for progress since it leads to comparisons of attitudes, sharing of expertise and exchange of ideas in a field where the techniques are evolving rapidly, as do cultural habits. Finally, progress and new techniques may solve or displace some ethical problems, as, for example, the case of intracytoplasmic sperm injection replacing donor insemination

107

when feasible: the difficult decisions implied in the relinquishing of the male genetic message in the couple may be displaced by other difficult decisions concerning a technique which is both more onerous physically on the female and financially to the couple or state.

But two factors still constitute an obstacle to better mutual understanding for all concerned – patients, practitioners and society at large. The first is the nature of the status of both embryo and fetus. Several countries have implemented psychosocial changes towards the recognition of a specific status for both these entities, mostly by means of an evolution of statutory law and court decisions. The status of both embryo and fetus is quite different from that of the born person. This leads to the acceptance of a 'third entity' besides the two categories of 'things' and 'persons' inherited from the particularly influential Roman law model in continental Europe. The second factor is more general and concerns relationships between 'patients' (or 'healthcare consumers') and the medical profession (or 'healthcare providers'). Here also diversity is striking. In a field where so many requests are linked to 'lifestyle choices', the respective roles and duties of the medical adviser or provider, and of the public authority responsible for allocation of scarce societal resources may significantly differ from one country to another.

Nevertheless, it may be stated that this diversity is more than compensated for by the conscience of the common goals shared by ART specialists. These common goals have been expressed very clearly in Article 2 of the Oviedo Convention (4.4.1997): 'the interests of the human being must prevail over those of science and society'. This has powerful implications to all of us who consider infertility a disease with painful consequences and which has to be regarded in the same way as any other disease.

Most societies also agree that a conscience clause concerning the possible handling of or research on the preimplantation embryo needs to apply to practitioners who do not wish to be involved. This clause is symmetrical to the patient's fundamental right of choice. But there is no such harmony when it comes to sociopolitical decisions about public funding of the cost of infertility treatments, especially in the case of specific requests (as in the treatment of single women for instance). Last but certainly not least, what is specific to infertility treatments is the need to take account of the welfare of future children born from ART, and more generally to consider the interests of future generations. These interests are first linked to the safety of the techniques and to the health of the children: lack of risk of transmitted viral or other diseases and safety with regard to the transmission of genetic disorders. Again there is general agreement in Europe about this responsibility and the need for effective preventive measures to be incorporated into guidelines, if not legislation. Many agree also that effective and careful follow-up of ART children is needed to increase safety and welfare for future generations.

At the same time we are convinced that future generations also have strong interests, if not rights, to benefit from the progress of science, technology and research in reproductive medicine. Thus when so many patients already benefit from research and innovative practice performed decades ago by Edwards and Steptoe, it would be unacceptable to hinder further progress by imposing too strict a legal framework, unless the reasons are overwhelming. It must be acknowledged that this position entails the acceptance of embryo and gametes research.

One may again expect to find polarized attitudes, but one should note that the evolution of the ethical analysis of ART dilemmas has been fairly rapid in the last 20 years, reflecting that of science. It is unlikely to slow down in the future.

Index